Cardiac

Dysrhythmia Interpretation

Workbook

New to the eighth edition of this workbook are th
These codes, as seen below, link to websites or v
or tablet computer with a camera you can downlc
hold the scanner over top of the code it will take v
on that page of the book such as a webpage witl

Paramedic Tutor Blog:
http://paramedictutor.wordpress.com
Videos links are under the eLearner tab

Paramedic Tutor YouTube Channel:
http://goo.gl/mcbJY

Eighth Edition

Rob Theriault BHSc., EMCA, RCT(Adv.), CCP(F)

West Sussex Knowledge & Libraries

Copy Number   CR 2160345

Table of contents

Introduction

This workbook was written with the intent of providing learners with a basic overview of cardiac anatomy, physiology, electrophysiology and electrocardiogram (ECG) interpretation. As a *workbook*, it is designed to assist you in reviewing the information covered in a dysrhythmia (arrhythmia) interpretation course.

Learning to interpret ECGs is a game of searching for clues and evidence that will lead you to an accurate interpretation. It can be fun and easy when you learn to use a systematic approach. Like any other skill, it needs to be used often it will be retained.

At this point it is worth mentioning that one of the downfalls some health care professionals experience soon after learning to interpret ECGs is a tendency to focus on the cardiac monitor and to forget about the patient.

REMEMBER: The cardiac monitor is an adjunct to your patient assessment and does not negate the need for assessing your patient's overall clinical status (i.e. assessing the patient's level of distress, level of awareness, taking a pulse, measuring the blood pressure, auscultating the chest, etc.).

Learning Outcomes

Upon completion of the book and the course with which this book is used, the learner will able to:

- Identify basic structures of the heart
- Describe the basic functions of the heart
- Describe the basic electrophysiology of cardiac contractile and conduction cells
- Compare and contrast ECG waves (electrical) with the heart's pumping (mechanical) activity
- List the common bipolar leads and certain special leads used in cardiac monitoring and identify the location of the lead placements
- interpreting cardiac dysrhythmias using a _step by step_ approach
- recognize life-threatening dysrhythmias

Part 1

CARDIAC *Anatomy, Physiology & Electrophysiology*

Cardiac Anatomy, Physiology & Electrophysiology

Outline

Anatomy:

- ♥ cardiac anatomy
- ♥ conduction system

Physiology:

- ♥ blood flow through the heart
- ♥ contractility
- ♥ Starling's law

ELECTROPHYSIOLOGY

- ♥ automaticity
- ♥ rhythmicity
- ♥ conductivity
- ♥ intercalated discs
- ♥ functional syncytium
- ♥ refractory period
- ♥ external influences: Autonomic nervous system

Cardiac Anatomy

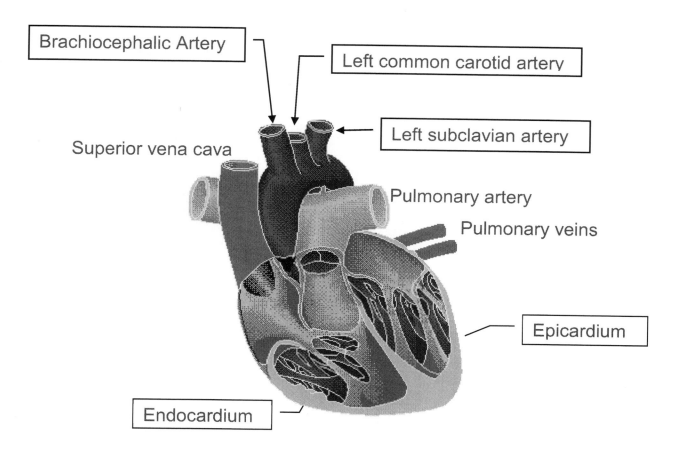

Brachiocephalic Artery

Left common carotid artery

Superior vena cava

Left subclavian artery

Pulmonary artery

Pulmonary veins

Epicardium

Endocardium

Rings that support the valves of the heart.

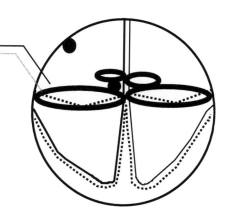

Surrounding the atrioventricular (AV) valves and the pulmonic and aortic valves are fibrous connective tissue rings. These rings not only provide support for the valves, but they effectively isolate the atria from the ventricles electrically. In the normal heart, the only electrical link between the atria and the ventricles is the AV node and Bundle of His.

Cardiac
Anatomy, Physiology & Electrophysiology

From your past anatomy & physiology classes you might recall the heart being described in the following way: The heart is a four chambered, *two sided* pump. The right side of the heart receives blood that has made its way through the body and is now returning after supplying the body with the necessary oxygen and nutrients needed to survive and thrive. This returning blood is now low in oxygen (O_2) and laden with carbon dioxide (CO_2) which is a waste product of metabolism. The blood enters the right atrium via the superior and inferior vena cava. And, blood from the heart muscle itself returns to the right atrium via the coronary sinus. From the right atrium, blood flows passively through the tricuspid valve into the right ventricle. The right ventricle receives approximately 70% of its volume passively, at which point the right atrium contracts, propelling the remaining 30% volume into the ventricle. The right ventricle then contracts, propelling the blood through the pulmonic valve, into the pulmonary artery where it travels *a very short distance* to the lungs. There, the blood gives off CO_2 to the atmosphere and takes in O_2.

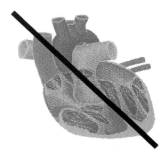

> From an anatomical perspective, we look at the heart as a four chambered, two sided pump – the right and left side.

Because the right ventricle pumps blood a short distance, it is a comparatively thin walled chamber.

After the blood has made its way through the pulmonary circulation, the now oxygen enriched blood returns to the left atrium via the pulmonary veins. The blood enters the left atrium and flows passively through the mitral valve into the left ventricle. The Like the right ventricle, the left receives approximately 70% of its volume passively, at which point the left atrium contracts, propelling the remaining 30% volume into the ventricle. The left ventricle then contracts, propelling the blood a *much greater distance* to all the organs and tissues, thus its thinker musculature. Once the blood reaches the tissue level CO2 diffuses from the tissues to the blood and O_2 is released from hemoglobin and diffuses to the tissues.

Myocardial cells

Cardiac muscle cells are similar in appearance to skeletal muscle cells in that they are striated (striped). However, skeletal muscle fibers are relatively long, contain many nuclei and are under voluntary control. Whereas, cardiac muscle fibers are much smaller, contain only one nucleus per cell and fall under the smooth (involuntary) muscle group.

The cells of the heart possess a number of valuable properties which allow them to perform their special function. These properties are:

Automaticity / Autorhyhmicity

The heart is the only organ that has this remarkable ability to generate impulses spontaneously – i.e. without the "need" for external stimulation from the nervous system. This is a property known as automaticity or autorhythmicity.

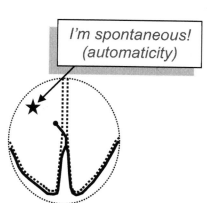

I'm spontaneous!
(automaticity)

Virtually any cell or group of cells within the myocardium is capable of producing impulses. However certain cells, known as *pacemaker cells,* are inherently better at generating spontaneously impulses than others. A basic principle dictates that the *pacemaker* site that fires the fastest controls the heart rate. In the healthy heart, the group of cells that fires the fastest and acts as the heart's intrinsic pacemaker is the sinoatrial (SA) node. Located in the right upper hand corner of the right atrium just below the entrance of the *superior vena cava*, the SA node normally fires at 60-80 beats (impulses) per minute in adults, but is capable of slower and faster rates in order to meet the changes in the body's metabolic demands.

If for some reason the SA node fails to generate impulses (or "pace" the heart), either due to disease, ischemia, infarction or other cause, back-up pacemaker sites such as those of the atrioventricular (AV) junction or the Purkinje system may assume the role of pacing the heart. These sites are referred to as "escape pacemaker" sites and serve as a backup system if the SA node fails.

Rhythmicity

When impulses are generated from a single location, known as a focus (the focus may be the SA node or any other location), they tend to fire RHYTHMICALLY. Irregularities in the heart's rhythm arise when there are competing foci (e.g. atrial fibrillation, premature ventricular complexes, etc...to be discussed later) or when there are disturbances in conduction (e.g. certain heart blocks). The concept of rhythmicity becomes important when trying to differentiate between some dysrhythmias.

Conduction system

Throughout the heart are groups of specialized cells that form the heart's conduction system. They are electrical fibers that weave their way through the myocardium carrying impulses rapidly to the contractile cells. This allows for coordinated contractions of the atria and ventricles. See page 12.

Conductivity

This refers to the cell's ability to transmit impulses to adjacent cells causing a spread of electrical current that is much like a domino effect. Cells that make up the heart's conduction system carry the spread of electrical current at a higher

speed (*conduction velocity*) than the contractile cells. Thus, the conduction system winds its way through the heart much like a rapid transit system carrying its passengers to their place of work, the muscles.

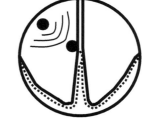

Someone once said, rather eloquently, that the waves of current that spread from the impulses of the SA node are like the wave in a pond from a pebble.

Like pebbles in a pond

Intercalated disks

Unique to cardiac muscle, these dark bands located where cardiac cells join end to end on the plasma membrane are specialized regions called "gap junctions". These intercalated disks allow impulses to travel very rapidly from cell to cell in a coordinated fashion.

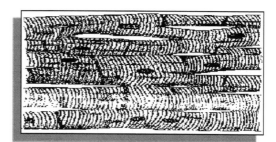

Intercalated Disks

Functional syncytium

Because of the presence of intercalated disks between cardiac cells and the speed with which impulses are conducted from cell to cell, the heart has been described as a group of cells working as one. This is the property of functional syncytium.

Contractility

Contractility is the ability of myocardial cells to respond to an impulse by contracting.

Starling's law

Within physiological limits, the more cardiac muscle fibers are stretched, the greater their force of contraction. Fully stretched, the heart can pump as much as five times its normal volume of blood. This allows the heart to respond to increased demands during exercise or stress.

Refractory period

This is a period during which the heart or part of the heart is unable to respond to an impulse. Cardiac muscle fibers must recover and return to a polarized state before they can depolarize and contract again.

"NO MUSCLE WORKS HARDER, LONGER OR MORE STEADILY."

Conduction System

When one cell depolarizes, cells adjacent to it are stimulated to depolarize.

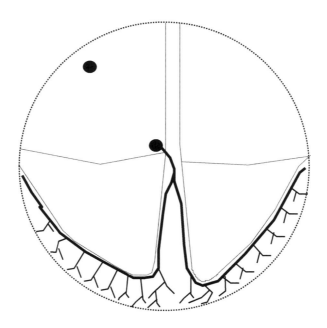

Electrophysiology: The impulse is born in the SA node and initiates a wave of depolarization across the atria.

The wave of depolarization travels across the atria via inter-nodal pathways until it reaches the AV node. There, the wave (impulse) is slowed to allow time for the atria to contract and expel their content into the ventricles. Once the impulse emerges from the AV node, it picks up speed down the Bundle of His. From there the conduction system bifurcates, forming the right and left bundle branches along which the impulse reaches its final destination in the Purkinje fibers.

The conduction system of the heart is like a rapid transit system that carries the message of electrical current to the contractile cells.

Conduction system: Inherent heart rates

SA Node   :   60-80   beats/minute (*average*)
AV Node   :   40-60   beats/minute
Purkinje system: 20-40   beats/minute

SA Node: 60-80 beats\min ⟶

AV Junction: 40-60 beats/min ⟶

Purkinje Fibers: 20-40 beats/min.

Conduction cells
- Those that generate impulses, i.e. pacemaker cells.
- Those that conduct impulses (like a rapid transit system).
- Impulses travel through the conduction system at 1 meter/sec., or 2-4 times faster than through contractile cells.

Myocardial cells
- Contractile element of the heart.
- Can generate *ectopic* impulses.

Definition: An ectopic impulse is one that originates in any part of the heart other than the SA node (primary pacemaker).

Electrophysiology
at the cellular level

How impulses form and how they conduct

Initiation and conduction of impulses result primarily from the exchange of three ions across the cell membrane: Sodium (Na^+), calcium (Ca^{++}) and potassium (K^+). This movement of electrolytes is represented by the "action potential" which is essentially a measurement of the electrical current of the cell. It's like an electrocardiogram of a single cell.

Polarized State. In the cell's resting state, K^+ is concentrated mainly on the inside of the cell, while Na^+ is concentrated mainly on the outside. The inside of the cell has a relatively negative charge compared with the outside due to the presence of other ions inside the cell that are negatively charged (anions) as well as the presence of non-diffusible proteins which act like anions. *The resting cell is said to be polarized* because the number of negative charges on the inside is equal to the number of positive charges on the outside. This *polarized state* is also known as the *resting membrane potential*.

Depolarization. When the cell becomes stimulated by an electrical impulse the cell becomes more permeable to Na^+. Na^+ migrates quickly into the cell, making the cell more positive on the inside. This generates electrical current and is the process known as *depolarization.* **Depolarization of muscle cells results in contraction**. During depolarization and in the early phase of the cell's recovery, there is also a slow influx of Ca^{++}. Calcium, in addition to assisting in the generation of electrical current (electrical element), is also the electrolyte needed for muscle contraction (mechanical element).

Repolarization. After the cell has depolarized, it begins down the road toward *repolarization*, or the return of the cell to its resting state. Immediately following depolarization the fast Na^+ channel closes. This is followed by a dip in the action potential resulting from a small efflux of K^+ (phase 1). After this small dip in the action potential the cell enters a "plateau' phase where there is an influx of Ca^{++} and little change in the membrane potential. Repolarization begins when there is another efflux of K^+ resulting in the downward slope of the action potential toward the baseline. Then the Na^+/K^+ pumps, located on the cell membrane, begin to return Na^+ and K^+ to their place of origin. This completes the return of the cell to the resting membrane potential. The Na^+/K^+ pump requires energy and is therefore an *active transport* process moving Na^+ out of the cell and K^+ back into the cell. **So once again, K^+ is concentrated on the inside of the cell while Na^+ is concentrated on the outside.** See pages 14 and 22.

Electrophysiology
at the cellular level

There are two fundamental types of cardiac cells

Muscle cells (contractile element)   Conduction cells (electrical element)

Although impulses travel 2-4 times faster through conduction cells than muscle cells, the electrical behaviour of both types of cells is essentially the same. To understand how impulses are conducted through the heart, we need only look at a single cells.

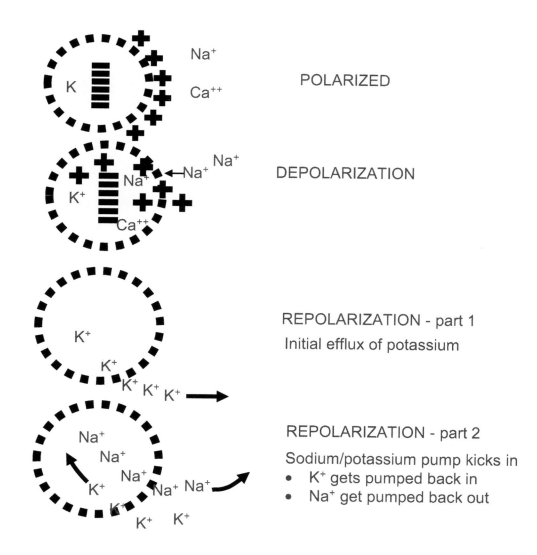

POLARIZED

DEPOLARIZATION

REPOLARIZATION - part 1

Initial efflux of potassium

REPOLARIZATION - part 2

Sodium/potassium pump kicks in
- K^+ gets pumped back in
- Na^+ get pumped back out

Autonomic Nervous System

Earlier, we discussed automaticity; the heart's ability to generate impulses without external influences. Now, let's look at the systems that affect the heart's performance.

The autonomic nervous system has two divisions, the *parasympathetic* and *sympathetic nervous systems.* Together they function in a "check-and-balance" manner to meet the metabolic demands of the body. They do so by influencing the rate of impulse formation, the speed of impulse conduction, and the strength of the heart's contraction. When the metabolic demands of the body are high, as they would be during exercise, the *sympathetic nervous system* dominates, increasing the heart rate and force of cardiac contraction. Conversely, when the body is at rest and the metabolic demands are low, the *parasympathetic nervous system* brings the heart rate and force of contraction down to a level that is appropriate to meet the body's needs.

Parasympathetic	Sympathetic
Slows it down	*Speeds it up*
Rest & Digest	*Fight or Flight*
↓ the heart rate	↑ the heart rate
↓ conduction velocity	↑ conduction velocity
↓ the force of contraction	↑ the force of contraction
mediated by the *vagus* nerve neurotransmitter: Acetylcholine	mediated by sympathetic nerves neurotransmitter: Epinephrine & norepinephrine

Some receptors you should be familiar with...

Parasympathetic division Receptors	Sympathetic division Receptors	Pertinent terminology
Nicotinic receptors: Located in skeletal muscle Muscurinic receptors: Located in smooth muscle STIMULATION Bronchi: Constriction, increased secretion Heart: ↓ heart rate Pupils: Pupillary constriction GI tract: ↑ peristalsis, ↑ secretions Salivary glands: ↑ salivation	Alpha 1 Located in vascular smooth muscle. Stimulation results in vasoconstriction. Alpha 2 Located in the CNS Stimulation results in peripheral vasodilation (e.g. certain antihypertensives) Beta 1 (one heart) Located in the heart. ↑ heart rate, ↑conduction, ↑contractility. Beta 2 (two lungs) Located in the smooth muscle of the bronchi and skeletal blood vessels. Bronchodilation, vasodilation. Dopaminergic In coronary, cerebral, renal and mesenteric vessels.	Chronotrope A substance that affects the heart rate. +ve chronotrope = ↑ heart rate -ve chronotrope = ↓ heart rate Inotrope A substance that affects myocardial contractility. +ve inotrope = ↑ force of contraction -ve inotrope = ↓ force of contraction Dromotrope Affects AV conduction velocity +ve dromotrope = ↑ AV conduction -ve dromotrope = ↓ AV conduction

Part 2

The

Electrocardiogram

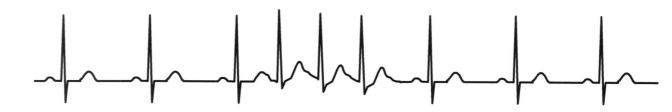

Electrocardiogram

Outline

ECG waves
- ♥ definition of the electrocardiogram
- ♥ ECG waves - What they represent
- ♥ ECG & its relation to cardiac contraction
- ♥ the action potential
- ♥ terms you should be familiar with

ECG Leads
- ♥ the common ECG monitoring Leads
- ♥ electrode placement
- ♥ where the Leads go
- ♥ MCL I Lead
- ♥ QRS deflection - Lead placement

Electrocardiogram: Definition

*The ECG represents the heart's **electrical** activity. The cardiac monitor senses this activity by means of disposable electrodes that are placed on the skin surface. The signal travels from the heart to the monitor where it is amplified and transcribed onto graph paper. The electrocardiogram will also sense skeletal muscle activity so it's important to avoid placing the electrodes over large muscle mass and to encourage the patient to lay still.*

Note: the abbreviation EKG, instead of ECG, is sometimes used to avoid confusion between ECG and EEG or to be faithful to the German origin of the EKG.

Electrocardiogram: What the ECG Waves Represent

P wave: Atrial depolarization (followed by atrial contraction)

QRS complex: Ventricular depolarization (followed by ventricular contraction)

T wave: Ventricular repolarization - return to the resting state

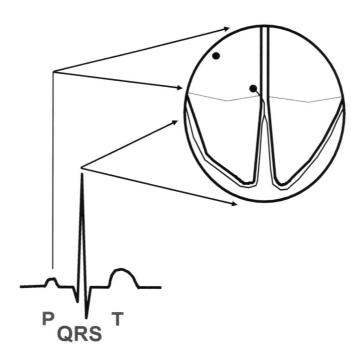

What do the ECG waves represent ?

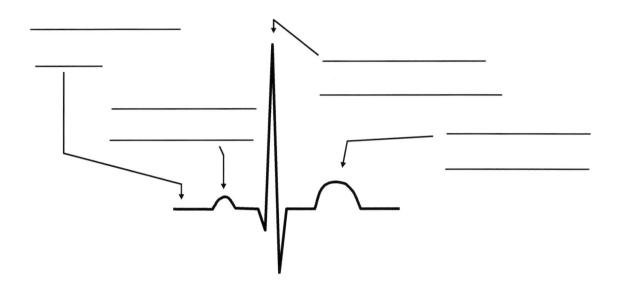

Notes:

_____

_____

_____

_____

_____

_____

_____

_____

_____

_____

_____

Electrocardiogram
in detail

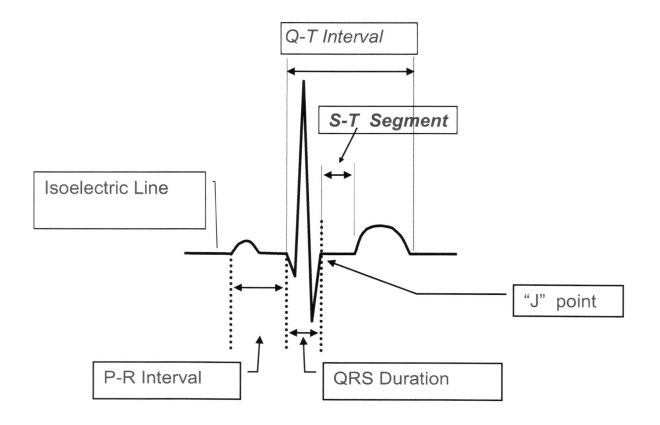

Q-T Interval

S-T Segment

Isoelectric Line

"J" point

P-R Interval

QRS Duration

Notes:

Action Potential

A graphic representation of the electrical activity of a single cell

The macroscopic/microscopic view

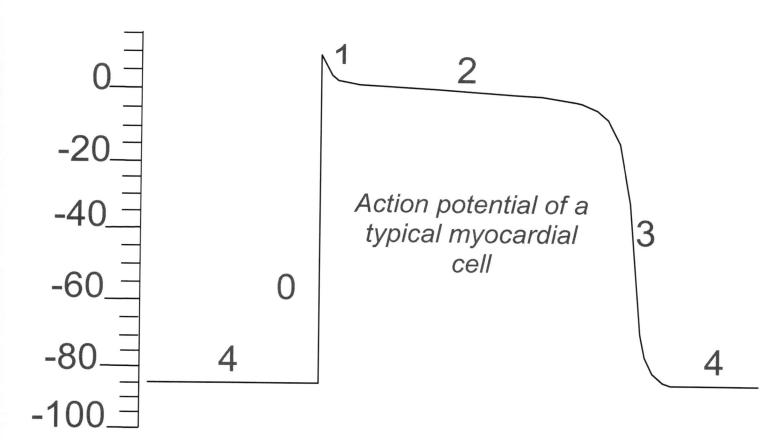

Action potential of a typical myocardial cell

Notes:

_____

_____

_____

_____

_____

_____

_____

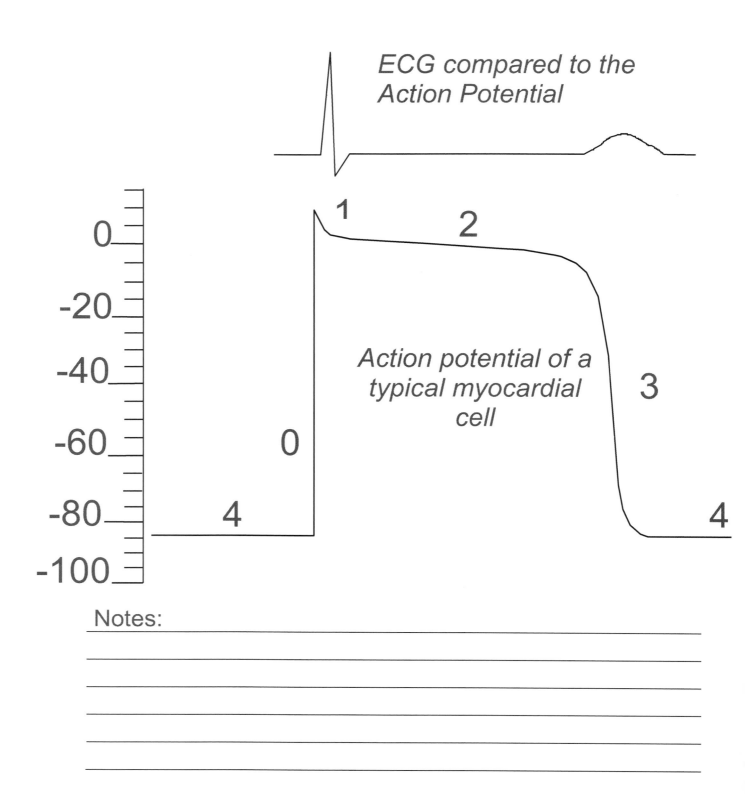

ECG compared to the Action Potential

Action potential of a typical myocardial cell

Notes:

Quick quiz: What do the following phases represent?

Phase 4: _____

Phase 0: _____

Phase 1: _____

Phase 2: _____

Phase 3: _____

Notes: _____

_____

_____

_____

_____

_____

_____

_____

_____

Action potential of a pacemaker cell

Threshold, or the point at which rapid depolarization occurs, takes place at approximately -ve 60.

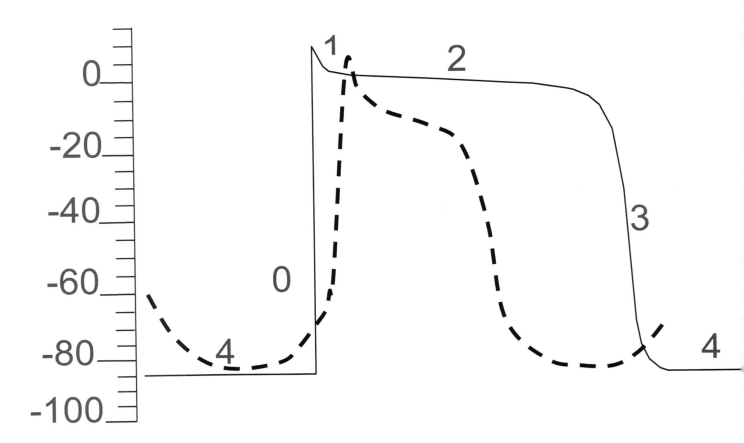

Notes:

_____

_____

_____

_____

_____

_____

_____

Terms you should be familiar with...

Cardiac cycle: *The interval from the beginning of one heart beat to the next. On the ECG, the cardiac cycle begins at the P wave and ends at the next PQRST or from one R wave to the next. The cardiac cycle includes systole and diastole.*

Absolute Refractory Period: *Begins at the onset of the QRS and continues until the peak of the T wave. It is the period during which the heart will not respond to another impulse.*

Relative Refractory Period: *On the ECG this is the brief period from the peak of the T wave through the downslope. It is the period during which the heart may be depolarized if a sufficiently strong impulse is generated. This is sometimes referred to as the "vulnerable" period because if as premature ventricular complex occurs at this time (called R on T phenomena) it may precipitate additional ectopic beats or short runs of ventricular tachycardia.*

Systole: *Is the contraction of the myocardium. Electrical systole refers to depolarization and begins at phase 0 and ends at phase 3 of the action potential.*

Diastole: *The relaxation phase of the heart. It is represented by phase 4 of the action potential (exception: pacemaker cell).* **It is during diastole that the coronary vessels receive their blood supply (perfusion takes place)**.

Heart Rate (HR): *The number of heart beats per minute. On the ECG it is the number of QRS complexes in one minute.*

Stroke Volume (SV): *The amount of blood ejected with each contraction of the left ventricle.*

Cardiac Output (CO): *The amount of blood pumped by the left ventricle for each minute. Cardiac output is calculated by multiplying heart rate by the stroke volume.*

CO = H.R. x Stroke volume

Terms continued...

Cardiac cycle

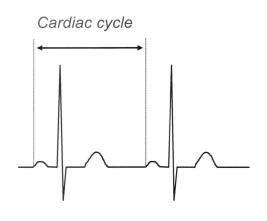

Absolute Refractory Period

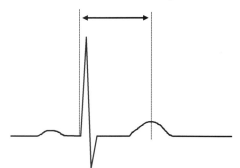

Relative Refractory Period
Vulnerable phase

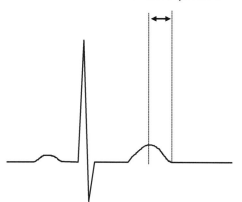

Ventricular systole

Atrial systole

Diastole

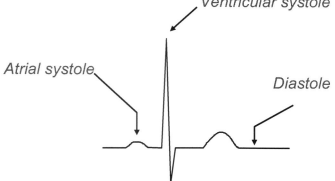

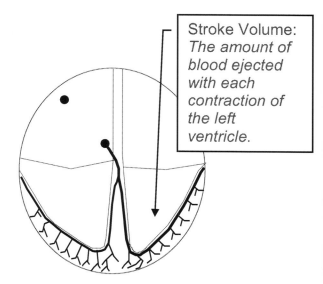

Stroke Volume:
The amount of blood ejected with each contraction of the left ventricle.

ECG LEADS

Einthoven's

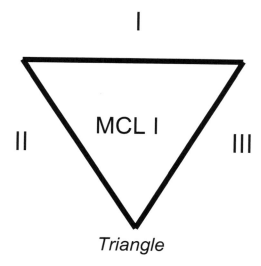

Triangle

Trivia: The first electrocardiogram on man was performed by Waller in 1887. The complexes recorded however were too small to be of any use.

Willem Einthoven, who is considered the Father of cardiology, is credited with modifying a device called the galvanometer which enabled him to obtain an accurate and interpretable representation of the heart's electrical activity. Modern electrocardiography was described by Einthoven in two papers that he published in 1907 and 1908.

Electrode placement

1. Make sure the skin surface is dry. Wipe the skin with a towel or alcohol swab if necessary. Sweaty or dirty skin will result in poor electrode contact and reduce the quality of the tracing.

2. Check the ECG electrodes on the under-surface to see that they are not dry or have ;ost their adhesive quality. A dry pad indicates that the electrode is old or has been exposed to air and will not sense the cardiac signal well.

3. Attach the ECG cables to the electrodes, then apply the electrodes to the skin surface using light pressure around the adhesive area.

4. To avoid artifact, do not place the electrodes over large muscle mass, bony protuberances, a pacemaker or implanted cardioverter-defibrillator.

5. Snap-on or clip-on lead cables are most commonly used in monitoring. Check the cables to ensure wires are not exposed or frayed.

Where the Leads go

The leads most commonly used in cardiac monitoring are the bipolar leads, leads I, II and III. They are called bipolar because they record the difference in electrical potential between two extremities (limbs). MCL I is another monitoring lead which is often used in the critical care setting (described further on).

Lead I

Records the difference in electrical voltage between the **right** and **left arm** . *The right arm electrode is negative . The left arm electrode is positive.*

Lead II

Records the difference in voltage between the **right arm** and the **left leg**.
The right arm electrode is negative .
The left leg electrode is positive .

Lead III

Records the difference in voltage between the **left arm** and the **left leg**.
The left arm electrode is negative. The left leg electrode is positive.

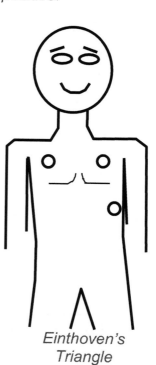

Einthoven's Triangle

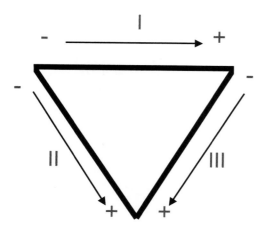

Where the Leads go

Leads are usually either <u>color coded</u> and/or marked with the first letters of the limb where they should be placed. i.e.. RA = right arm

e.g.   **RA** (white): Right arm electrode
       LA (black): Left arm electrode
       LL (red):   Left leg electrode

- White goes to the right.
- Red goes to the ribs.
- The color left over goes to the left shoulder.

Right arm electrode.
Typically placed on the right upper anterior chest just below the clavicle.
Alternative placement: right wrist, right shoulder, right upper scapula

Left arm electrode.
Typically placed on the left upper anterior chest just below the clavicle.
Alternative placement: left wrist, left shoulder, left upper scapula

Left leg electrode.
Typically placed on the left lateral chest wall, low enough so that it doesn't get in the way of placing the defibrillator pads (or paddles) or doing a twelve lead ECG.
Alternative placement: Left leg, left hip.

<u>Note</u>: *Many cardiac monitors have a fourth cable used exclusively as a ground lead. It can be placed anywhere on the body, but is most often placed on the right lateral chest wall or right leg.*

MCL I LEAD: a special Lead

Records the difference in voltage between the **left arm** and the **anterior chest**. *Left arm is negative. The chest lead is positive. The positive electrode is placed in the fourth intercostal space at the right sternal border* (same position as V1 in a 12 lead ECG).

MCL I: Modified chest lead I

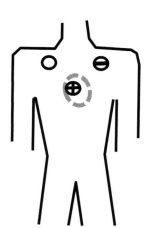

Placement

Turn *lead select* dial on the monitor to lead III.
The electrodes are placed as they would be normally, with one exception:
The LL (+ve) electrode is placed in the 4th intercostal space at the right sternal border (same position as V1 in a 12 Lead).

Purpose
MCL I highlights atrial activity by bringing out the P wave. It is able to do this because the +ve electrode sits close to the atria. MCL I is a good lead to use when it is difficult to discern P waves: e.g. narrow complex tachycardia, wide complex tachycardia where it is uncertain whether there is a wave preceding each QRS.

MCL I can also be used to determine whether a right or left bundle branch block exists or which ventricle an ectopic focus is coming from; although that is beyond the scope of this workbook.

QRS Deflection - Lead placement

Depolarization begins at the SA node and spreads toward the apex of the heart. If you summarize all the waves of depolarization you obtain a vector. Because the left ventricle is larger than the right, the vector is off to the left. Hence, the angle of the arrows in the diagrams below.

When a wave of depolarization moves toward a positive electrode there is a resulting positive (upward) QRS deflection recorded on the ECG, as illustrated in example A.

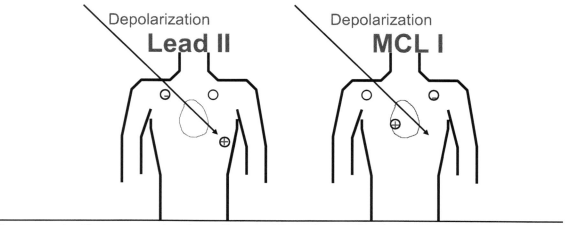

Conversely, if you were to place the positive electrode above the ventricles, as you would with an MCL I lead, the wave of depolarization moves away from the positive electrode resulting in a negatively (downward) deflected QRS; as seen in example B.

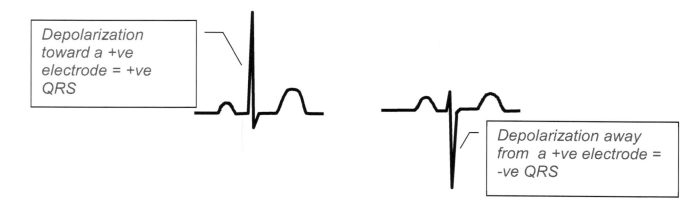

Depolarization toward a +ve electrode = +ve QRS

Depolarization away from a +ve electrode = -ve QRS

Part 3

CARDIAC DYSRHYTHMIA INTERPRETATION

Cardiac Dysrhythmia Interpretation

Outline

- ♥ ECG graph paper
- ♥ paper speed

- ♥ heart rate calculation
- ♥ ECG: intervals, durations & segments

- ♥ waves and complexes
- ♥ Step by Step approach
- ♥ Cardiac Rhythm Interpretation: Concepts

- ♥ rhythms and their descriptions

ECG GRAPH PAPER

To interpret rhythms, you need to know what the graph paper represents.

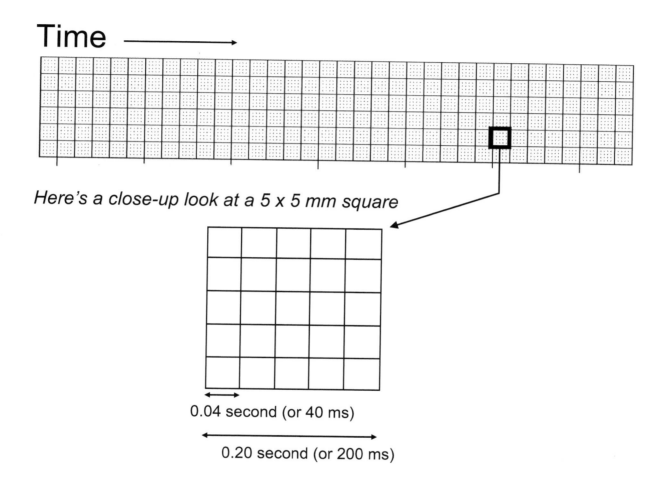

Time

Here's a close-up look at a 5 x 5 mm square

0.04 second (or 40 ms)

0.20 second (or 200 ms)

Paper speed
25 mm/second is the standard ECG paper speed.

Some monitors allow you to change the paper speed to 50 mm/sec. This widens the gap between the complexes and may make P waves more discernible in tachyarrhythmias where P waves sometimes get buried in the preceding T wave. This is sometimes used for ECG tracings in infants.

Heart rate calculation

Simple method – not very accurate

Count the number of QRS complexes in a six second strip and multiply by ten.
ECG graph paper will have markers at every one or three second interval.

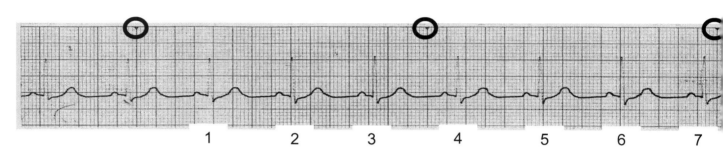

1   2   3   4   5   6   7

What is the heart rate? _____ x 10 = _____

Notes:

_____

_____

_____

_____

_____

_____

_____

_____

_____

_____

Heart rate calculation

Advanced method – more accurate

Rationale: The digital heart rate on a cardiac monitor can be inaccurate at times – especially when there is artifact present. Using a more accurate heart rate calculation method like the one below becomes critically important when the heart rate is excessively fast or very slow. Always verify the heart rate manually by using the following method:

1. Find an R wave that falls on a dark line.
2. Count the number of dark lines between neighboring R waves and divide into 300. Or, memorize the numbers below. It's worth the effort.

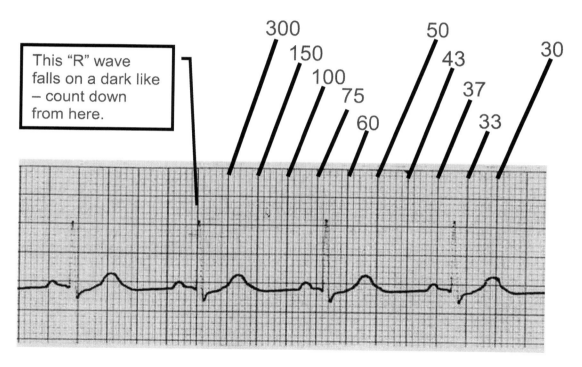

This "R" wave falls on a dark like – count down from here.

300
150
100
75
60
50
43
37
33
30

What would the heart rate would be if the second QRS fell between 300 and 150 or between 75 and 60. How much would each small square be worth?

Notes:

_____

_____

_____

Heart rate calculation practice

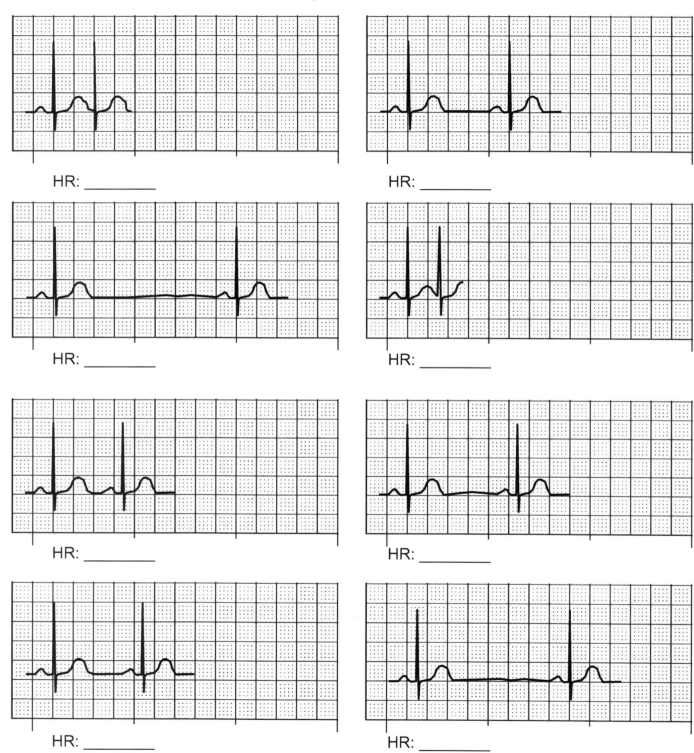

HR: _____

HR: _____

HR: _____

HR: _____

HR: _____

HR: _____

HR: _____

HR: _____

Waves and complexes

P Waves

- Represent atrial depolarization.
- P waves are normally upright in leads I, II and III.
- P waves may be contoured, notched or biphasic and still represent a sinus rhythm. The question you must ask yourself is: **_Are all the P waves the same shape?_**

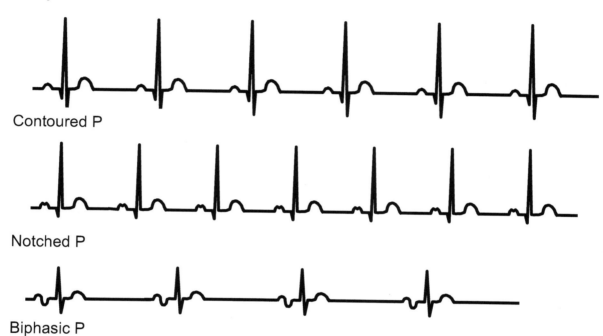

Contoured P

Notched P

Biphasic P

Notes:

_____

_____

_____

_____

_____

_____

P Waves - Junctional

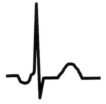

- Inverted P waves with short PR intervals suggest junctional rhythm.

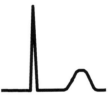

- Absent P waves followed by narrow QRS complexes also suggest a junctional rhythm.

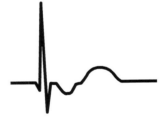

- Retrograde P waves (after the QRS) are suggestive of a junctional rhythm as well.

Notes:

_____

_____

_____

_____

_____

_____

_____

_____

P-R Interval

- the P-R interval represents the time it takes for the impulse to travel from the SA to the end of the Bundle of HIS.
- It is measured from the onset of the P wave until the onset of the QRS.
- A prolonged P-R interval, i.e. one > 0.20 second indicates there is a delay in conduction at the AV node or the perinodal tissues.

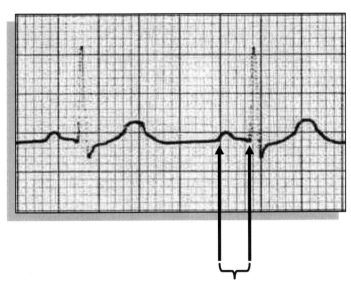

~ 4 small squares or
0.16 second

Other examples

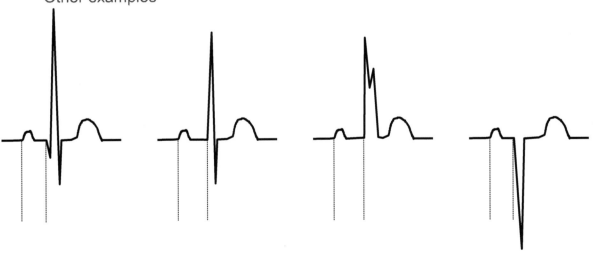

QRS Complexes

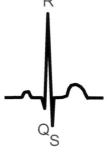

- Represent ventricular depolarization.
- Q wave: Is the first negative (downward) deflection.
- R wave: Is the first positive (upward) deflection.
- S wave: Is the second negative deflection.

- All three waves need not be present for it to be referred to as the QRS complex. When interpreting ECG rhythms, we are not interested in the QRS morphology (shape) or its deflection. We need only be concerned about the QRS duration. ***Are the QRSs narrow or wide?***

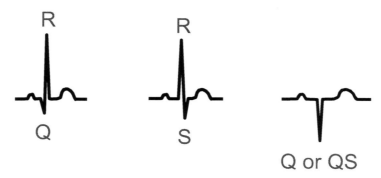

If the QRS is narrow, i.e. < 0.12 second, the impulse has to have traveled down both bundle branches simultaneously. If the QRS is wide, i.e. ≥ 0.12 second, then the impulse is either originating from a focus in one of the ventricles or it's coming from above the bifurcation of the bundle branches and is delayed in the ventricles.

T Waves

- Represent ventricular repolarization. Its morphology or deflection (vector) is not important where rhythm interpretation is concerned.

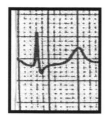
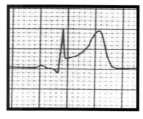
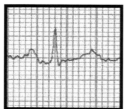
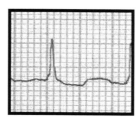
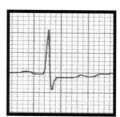

U Waves

- May represent the final stage of repolarization. A prominent U wave may suggest the presence of hypokalemia, cardiomyopathy, left ventricular hypertrophy or diabetes.

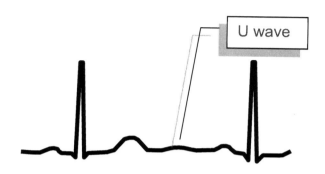

Notes:

STEP by STEP
APPROACH

RATE
What is the heart rate?

P WAVES
Are the P waves present? Are they regular? And, do they all look alike?
Are the P waves inverted, absent or retrograde: i.e.. a junctional rhythm?
Are there fibrillation or flutter waves?
Are the P waves buried and not clearly discernible?
Does artifact obscure the P waves?

PR INTERVAL
Is the PR interval equal or less than 0.20 second or is it prolonged (i.e. > 0.20 sec)?
If P waves are absent or not clearly discernible, then the PR interval is N/A.

QRS
Are the QRS complexes narrow (**< 0.12** sec.) or wide (**≥ 0.12** sec.)?

RATIO
Is there one P wave for every QRS (1:1 ratio), or is there more than 1:1, or is the ratio not applicable ?

Rhythm
Is the rhythm regular, regularly irregular or irregularly irregular?

Interpretation
Putting all the evidence together, describe the underlying rhythm, the rate and the disturbances.
e.g. Normal sinus rhythm of 74/min. with 8-10 PVCs per minute.

Note: *When describing an ECG rhythm, be sure to include the heart rate, as this is one of the determinants of cardiac output and may be the deciding factor on whether or how the patient is to be treated.*

Dysrhythmia Concepts

Now that you're familiar with the normal components of the ECG, it's time to look at disturbances in cardiac rhythm. Remember that when you are looking at rhythms on the monitor, you are *only* looking at the heart's *electrical* activity. Look at the rhythms and try to visualize the atria and the ventricles, electrically linked by the AV node and Bundle of His. With that in mind, ask yourself the following questions:

Is there atrial activity (P waves)? Is there ventricular activity (QRS)? Are the atria and ventricles working in sync with one another? i.e. is there one P wave for every QRS?

Is the distance between the P wave and the QRS normal? A prolonged P-R interval indicates a delay in conduction at the AV node, Bundle of HIS or the perinodal tissue.

Are impulses being generated by the heart's intrinsic pacemaker (the SA node) or are they being generated from some other site within the heart?

Are there ectopic beats? Do they originate in the atria or the ventricles?

These questions will help to guide you as you learn a systematic approach to cardiac dysrhythmia interpretation.

All dysrhythmias fall into one or both of the following categories:

Disorders in impulse formation
Impulses are *not* being formed where they should; i.e.. the SA node fails, either intermittently or permanently, or an impulse or impulses are generated elsewhere before the SA node is able to fire. When the SA node fails to fire and a back up pacemaker sites takes over the role, it is described as escape rhythm or escape pacemaker site. This is a compensatory response. The second disorder in impulse formation occurs when an ectopic focus fires an impulse before the next expected beat, as in a premature atrial complex (PAC) or a premature ventricular complex (PVC), or when an ectopic focus fires repetitively and faster than the SA node and takes over pacing of the heart – e.g. supraventricular tachycardia or ventricular tachycardia.

Disorders in impulse conduction
Impulses are delayed or blocked in some part of the heart. e.g. AV blocks

Reporting Dysrhythmias

Remember, *if you're describing the patient's condition to someone who is not at the patient's bed side, it is important to paint a complete and succinct picture. Describing the ECG rhythm alone is not enough. What is the heart rate? Are the patient's signs and symptoms attributable to the heart rate and/or rhythm? The physician at the receiving end of the report has to have a clear picture to make some decisions about rhythm and rate appropriate therapies.*

Notes:

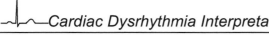

Normal sinus rhythm (NSR)

Example

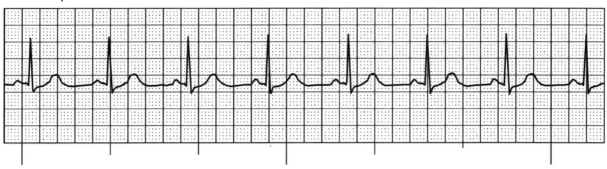

	Rate:	Heart rate is between 60 – 99
	P waves	Are present and upright in leads I, II and III.
	PR:	Normal, i.e. ≤ 0.20 second
	QRS:	Is usually narrow, i.e. < 0.12 second
	Ratio	1:1
	Rhythm:	Regular

Describe this rhythm: _____

In **NSR** the pacemaker site is the SA node.

The heart rate is between 60 - 99.

Remember that we do not care about the morphology of the QRS complex or T wave. A QRS of ≥ 0.12 second may suggest presence of an intraventricular conduction defect (IVCD). However that does not change our interpretation of the rhythm. **The QRS and T wave morphology have no impact on the rhythm interpretation.**

Sinus arrhythmia

Example

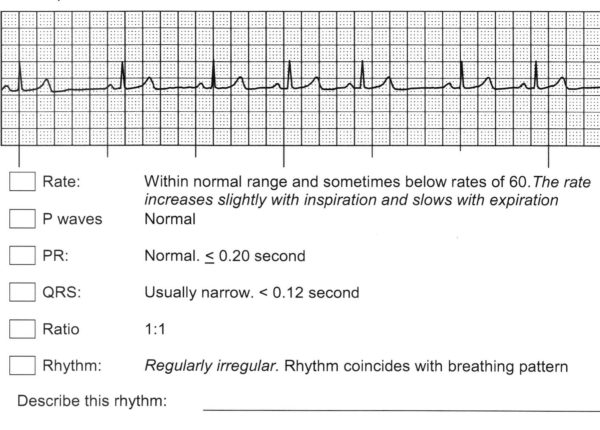

	Rate:	Within normal range and sometimes below rates of 60. *The rate increases slightly with inspiration and slows with expiration*
	P waves	Normal
	PR:	Normal. $\leq$ 0.20 second
	QRS:	Usually narrow. < 0.12 second
	Ratio	1:1
	Rhythm:	*Regularly irregular.* Rhythm coincides with breathing pattern

Describe this rhythm: _____

Sinus arrhythmia is considered a normal rhythm and is most commonly seen in children and young adults. The most common phasic (respiratory) variety is one where the rate increases with inspiration and decreases with expiration.

Inspiration decreases vagal tone resulting in a slight increase in heart rate and expiration restores vagal tone resulting in a decrease in heart rate (Bainbridge reflex). **No treatment is required.**

Heart rate varies slightly with the respiratory pattern

Sinus bradycardia

Example

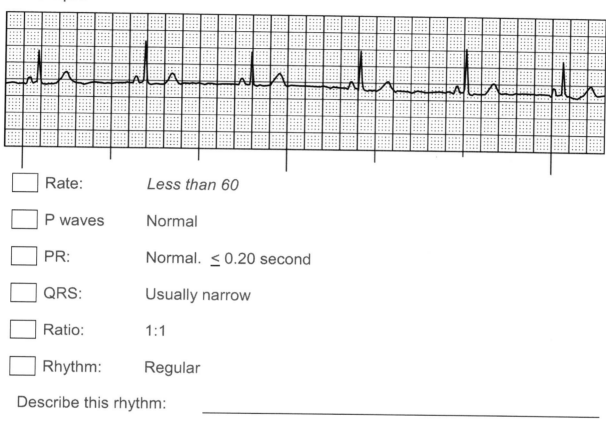

☐ Rate: *Less than 60*

☐ P waves   Normal

☐ PR: Normal. ≤ 0.20 second

☐ QRS: Usually narrow

☐ Ratio: 1:1

☐ Rhythm: Regular

Describe this rhythm: _____

_____

Sinus bradycardia results when the SA node fires at rates less than 60/min. It may be normal in athletes, while in others it may be the result of sinus node disease, an acute inferior wall infarction, increased vagal tone, hypothyroidism, raised intracranial pressure, or from the effects of certain drugs such as quinidine, beta blockers, or calcium channel blockers.

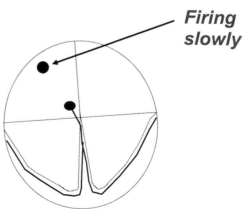

Firing slowly

Sinus tachycardia

Example

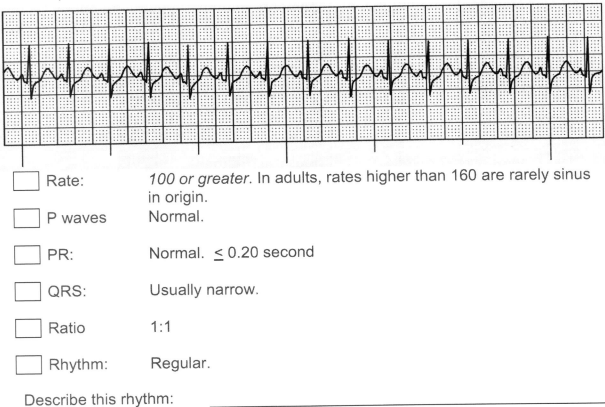

☐	Rate:	*100 or greater*. In adults, rates higher than 160 are rarely sinus in origin.
☐	P waves	Normal.
☐	PR:	Normal. ≤ 0.20 second
☐	QRS:	Usually narrow.
☐	Ratio	1:1
☐	Rhythm:	Regular.

Describe this rhythm: _____

_____

Sinus tachycardia results when the SA node fires at a rate equal or greater than 100/min. It is a normal response to increased metabolic demands placed on the body during exertion or a significant stress. It may also be caused by hypovolemia (reflex tachycardia), hypoxia, fever, pulmonary embolus, hyperthyroidism, etc.

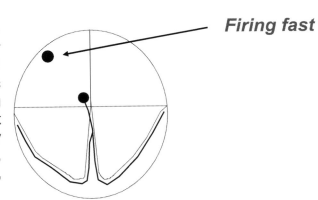

Firing fast

Supraventricular tachycardia (SVT)

Example

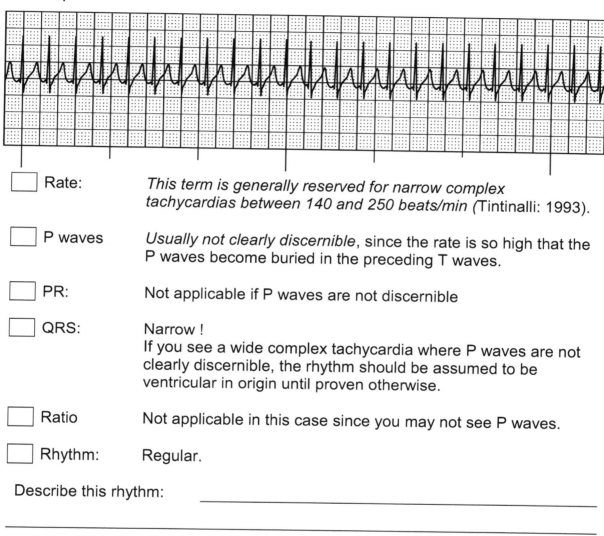

☐ Rate: *This term is generally reserved for narrow complex tachycardias between 140 and 250 beats/min (Tintinalli: 1993).*

☐ P waves   *Usually not clearly discernible,* since the rate is so high that the P waves become buried in the preceding T waves.

☐ PR: Not applicable if P waves are not discernible

☐ QRS: Narrow !
            If you see a wide complex tachycardia where P waves are not clearly discernible, the rhythm should be assumed to be ventricular in origin until proven otherwise.

☐ Ratio   Not applicable in this case since you may not see P waves.

☐ Rhythm: Regular.

Describe this rhythm: _____

_____

SVT may be due to some form of re-entry mechanism (discussed later). It is a catch-all term to describe regular narrow complex (QRS) tachyarrhythmias in which P waves *cannot clearly be seen*. If the QRS is narrow we know that the pacemaker site is somewhere above the bifurcation of the bundle branches and that both ventricles are depolarizing simultaneously.

Fast narrow complex tachycardia - Can't clearly make out P waves

Paroxysmal supraventricular tachycardia (PSVT)

Example

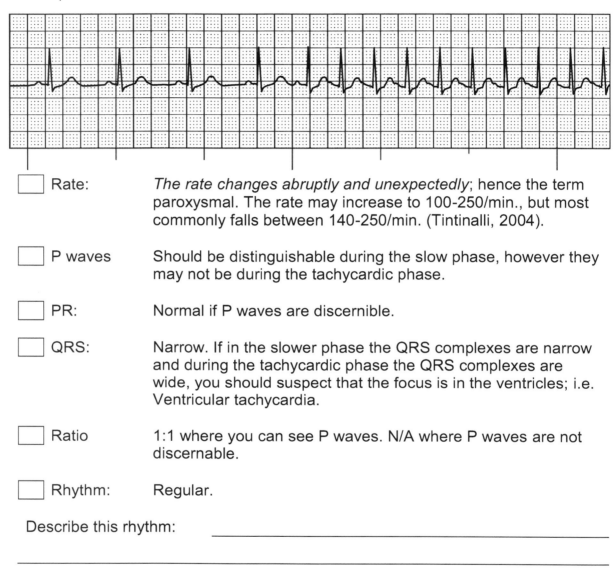

	Rate:	*The rate changes abruptly and unexpectedly*; hence the term paroxysmal. The rate may increase to 100-250/min., but most commonly falls between 140-250/min. (Tintinalli, 2004).
	P waves	Should be distinguishable during the slow phase, however they may not be during the tachycardic phase.
	PR:	Normal if P waves are discernible.
	QRS:	Narrow. If in the slower phase the QRS complexes are narrow and during the tachycardic phase the QRS complexes are wide, you should suspect that the focus is in the ventricles; i.e. Ventricular tachycardia.
	Ratio	1:1 where you can see P waves. N/A where P waves are not discernable.
	Rhythm:	Regular.

Describe this rhythm: _____

PSVT *continued*

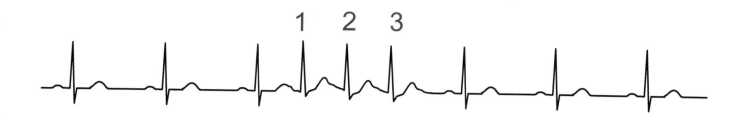

1   2   3

✓ Bouts of PSVT may be as short as three fast beats in a row

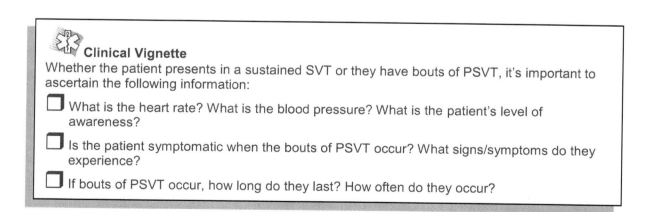

Clinical Vignette

Whether the patient presents in a sustained SVT or they have bouts of PSVT, it's important to ascertain the following information:

☐ What is the heart rate? What is the blood pressure? What is the patient's level of awareness?

☐ Is the patient symptomatic when the bouts of PSVT occur? What signs/symptoms do they experience?

☐ If bouts of PSVT occur, how long do they last? How often do they occur?

Causes of PSVT

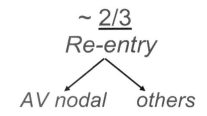

~ 2/3
Re-entry

AV nodal   others

Circus movement tachycardia at the microscopic level

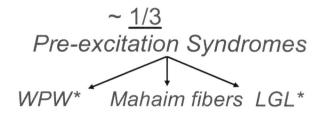

~ 1/3
Pre-excitation Syndromes

WPW   Mahaim fibers   LGL**

Circus movement tachycardia at the macroscopic level

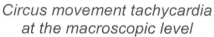

WPW

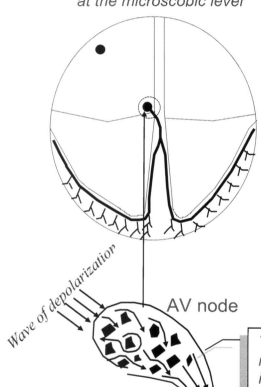

Wave of depolarization

AV node

The AV node is made up of patches of non-conductive tissue and interweaving and interconnecting fibers. This means that there is the potential for re-entry, as described on the following page

*WPW = Wolff-Parkinson-White Syndrome
*LGL = Lown-Ganong-Levine Syndrome

Re-entry

"Re-entry is a condition in which an impulse remains active in some part of the heart and reactivates the myocardium after the main impulse that spawned it has finished its route and the surrounding fibers have repolarized" (Conover: 1988). Re-entry occurs when an impulse deviates around a circular pathway or "loop".

In order for re-entry to occur, the following conditions are necessary:

1. A potential circular pathway.

2. A unidirectional block within part of that circuit.

3. Delayed conduction in the rest of the circuit.

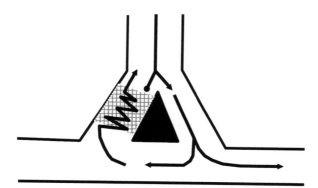

A wave of depolarization encounters a region that is non-conductive and deviates around it. Down the right limb, the wave of depolarization continues. Down the left limb, it encounters a group of cells that are still refractory and the wave is blocked.

The wave (impulse) of depolarization spreads to the rest of the heart causing it to contract and repolarize. Meanwhile, the previously blocked conduction limb is now able to conduct slowly in a retrograde direction.

Now the impulse re-enters a polarized or repolarizing region and gives rise to an ectopic focus that may generate a single beat or give rise to a series of consecutive beats as is seen in PSVT.

Pre-excitation syndromes

Wolff-Parkinson-White   Mahaim fibers   Lown-Ganong-Levine

Pre-excitation is a term used to describe a syndrome where an impulse from the atria reaches the ventricles sooner than it would be expected to if it were transmitted down the normal conduction pathway; i.e. via the AV node.

Normally, the atria and ventricles are electrically isolated from one another by fibrous connective tissue rings that support the AV valves and the aortic and pulmonic valves. The only electrical link between the atria and ventricles in the normal heart is the AV node and Bundle of His.

In some individuals, pre-excitation occurs because there exists a muscle fiber or accessory pathway that bypasses the AV node.

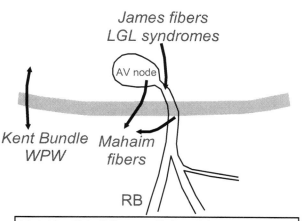

Adapted from Tintinalli: Emergency Medicine; A Comprehensive Study Guide; sixth Edition, New York: 2004

Wolff-Parkinson-White Syndrome: The Kent bundle is an accessory pathway that inserts into the ventricle and provides a conduction pathway that bypasses the AV node. Conduction is through the AV node then up from the ventricle to the atria by way of the accessory pathway in 80-95% of cases. In the remainder of cases, conduction is anterograde, or from the atria directly into the ventricle. If the ventricles are activated simultaneously through the AV node and the accessory pathway, the initial phase of the QRS complex is slurred, forming a "Delta wave".

Mahaim fibers: These originate in either the AV node, The HIS Bundle or the bundle branches. Impulses travel through the AV node, then into the ventricles through the accessory pathway(s) and the His bundle simultaneously.

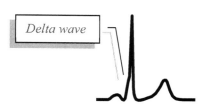

Lown-Ganong-Levine (LGL) Syndrome: Several structural anomalies have been proposed as the possible basis for LGL, including the presence of James fibers, Mahaim fibers, Brechenmacher-type fibers, and an anatomically underdeveloped (hypoplastic) or small AV node. James fibers run from the upper portion of the AV node and insert in the lower portion or in the bundle of His

Junctional rhythm

Example

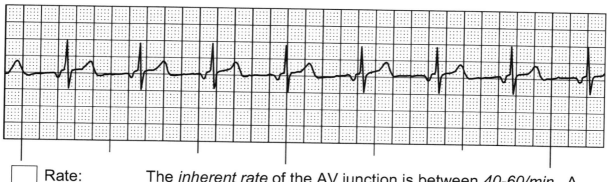

☐ **Rate:** The *inherent rate* of the AV junction is between *40-60/min.* A rate above 60 would be called: An accelerated junctional rhythm.

☐ **P waves** *Inverted, absent or retrograde* (occurring after the QRS).

☐ **PR:** Normal, short, or not applicable.

☐ **QRS:** Usually narrow.
Remember: If you don't see P waves and the QRS is wide, always assume the rhythm is ventricular because it usually is. If treatment is required, making the correct rhythm interpretation may be critical.

☐ **Ratio** 1:1 if P waves are present.

☐ **Rhythm:** Regular

Describe this rhythm: _____

_____

Junctional rhythms generally do not require treatment, unless the rate is markedly slow and the patient is symptomatic as a result.

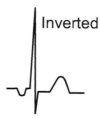 Inverted

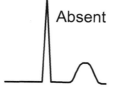 Absent

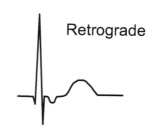 Retrograde

Premature atrial complex (PAC)

Example

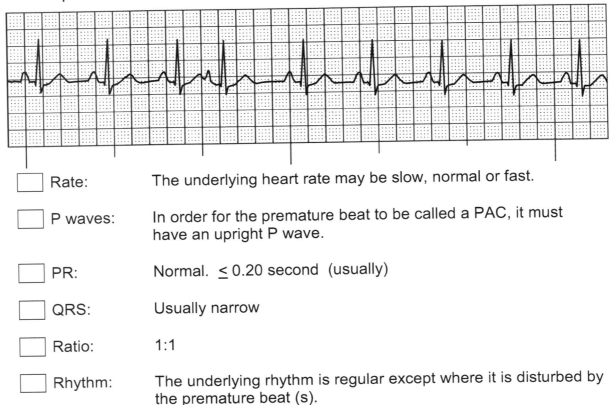

	Rate:	The underlying heart rate may be slow, normal or fast.
	P waves:	In order for the premature beat to be called a PAC, it must have an upright P wave.
	PR:	Normal. ≤ 0.20 second (usually)
	QRS:	Usually narrow
	Ratio:	1:1
	Rhythm:	The underlying rhythm is regular except where it is disturbed by the premature beat (s).

Describe this rhythm: _____

A PAC results from the firing of an ectopic impulse somewhere in the atria. It occurs prematurely or before the next expected beat. The P wave in a PAC may have a similar or different morphology from the P waves in the underlying rhythm. The P wave must however be upright to call it a PAC.

If the P wave is inverted or retrograde then it would be called a _premature junctional beat (PJC)_.

If you see a narrow complex premature beat where the P wave is not clearly discernible, you can use the catch-all term: _Supraventricular premature beat (SVPB)_.

Premature narrow complex beat with a P wave

PREMATURE BEATS
from above the ventricles

PJC

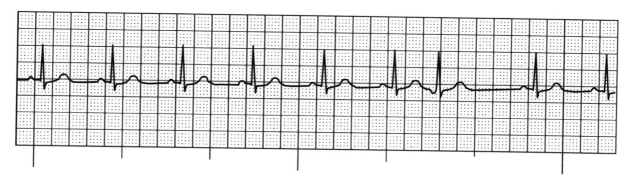

SVPB

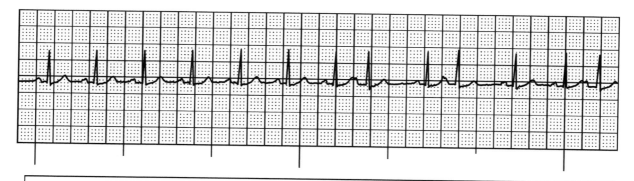

 Note

Supraventricular premature beat (SVPB) is a term used to describe a narrow [QRS] complex premature beat where it's difficult to determine the origin of the focus (if not obviously atrial or junctional). However, although it's worth being familiar with the term SVPB, it is not a term commonly used in the emergency setting.

Sinus arrest or pause

Example

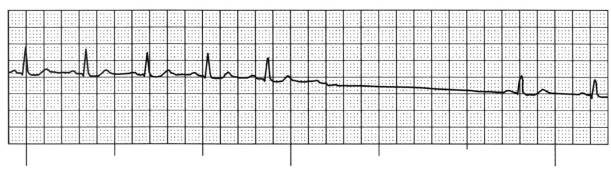

	Rate:	The underlying heart rate may be slow, normal or fast.
☐	P waves	Present and upright in the underlying rhythm. The P wave following the pause is frequently different in shape since it is likely to originate from an escape pacemaker site.
☐	PR:	Normal or prolonged.
☐	QRS:	Usually narrow.
☐	Ratio	1:1
☐	Rhythm:	The underlying rhythm is regular except where it is disturbed by the premature beat (s).

Describe this rhythm: _____

Sinus arrest is an example of a disorder in impulse formation. The SA node fails to generate an impulse for a prolonged period of time. The beat that occurs at the end of the pause typically originates from an area other than the SA node, is referred to as an *escape beat* and is compensatory in nature.

Fails to fire = cause of the pause

Sinus arrest is basically a brief episode of asystole and may lead to cardiac arrest if not treated promptly. Patients with this dysrhythmia are candidates for a pacemaker.

Sinus exit block

Example

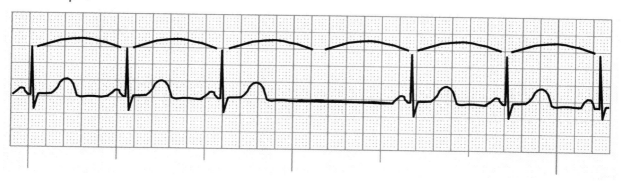

☐ Rate:	Slow to normal	
☐ P waves	Normal in the underlying rhythm.	
☐ PR:	Normal. ≤ 0.20 second (usually)	
☐ QRS:	Usually narrow.	
☐ Ratio	1:1	
☐ Rhythm:	Regular except where disrupted by the dropped beats.	

Describe this rhythm: _____

_____

In sinus exit block, or SA block, impulses are generated by the SA node but because of a disorder in impulse conduction *some cannot progress to the rest of the atria* since surrounding cells are still refractory. This may be due to disease or local ischemia.

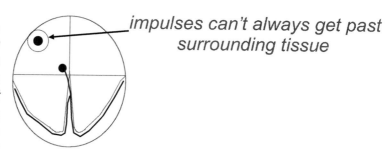

impulses can't always get past surrounding tissue

Where you see a dropped beat, the interval between beats is a multiple of the cardiac cycle, meaning that the next beat falls where you would expect it to; this is the distinction between *sinus exit block* and *sinus arrest*.

Atrial fibrillation

Example

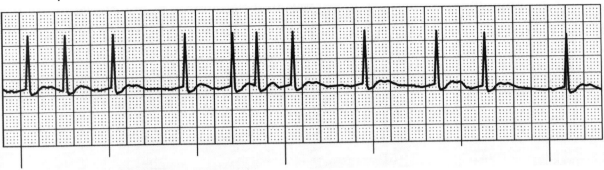

	Rate:	*Will vary.* When describing the rate in A. fib. we do so in terms of the ventricular response. e.g. atrial fib. with a ventricular response of 80-110.
	P waves	Multiple foci fire in the atria, none of which effectively depolarize the atria. On the ECG, the result is either an *uneven fibrillatory baseline or a flat line between QRSs.*
	PR:	N/A
	QRS:	Usually narrow. If you see a wide complex rhythm that is irregularly irregular and you cannot make out P waves, chances are you're dealing with A. fib. with an underlying bundle branch block.
	Ratio	N/A
	Rhythm:	*The hallmark of atrial fib. is that it is irregularly irregular* !!

Describe this rhythm: _____

_____

Atrial fibrillation, or A. Fib. occurs when multiple foci within the atria discharge randomly. The result is a multiple waves of depolarization that collide and cancel one another our resulting in a quivering mass of atrial myocardium. The atria **do not** contract. Despite this, 70% of the ventricle's blood volume is reached passively as blood returns to the heart via the vena cava and flows from the atria to the ventricles without the atria having to contract. The remaining blood volume, approximately 30 %, stays in the atria until the next cardiac cycle. This stasis of blood can result in the formation of micro clots. Hence the reason atrial fib. is one of the most common causes of embolic stroke. Emboli that form in the atria may also travel to, and block vessels in the pulmonary and mesenteric vascular bed.

In atrial fib., ectopic foci fire at a rate greater than 350/minute. Only a limited number of impulses are able to reach the ventricles thanks to the protection of the AV node.

Ectopic foci: Impulsive party animals that reek havoc on the chambers they seek to party in. A few of them are a mere irritation; a chamber full of them means chaos!

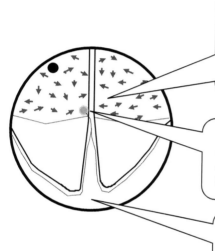

*Hey AV node! Us ectopics are feelin' **impulsive**. We have the urge to surge into the chambers down below where there's more room to party! We're already **irritable, so** don't slow us down!*

*Sorry party animals! Look at the mess you've made upstairs; you've turned the atria into a quivering mess. Besides, you know that every time I let one of you through, **I need my normal resting period**.*

Hey Node-man! You neglected to mention that when you let too many ectopics get through, I get very irritable!

 Clinical Vignette

When atrial fibrillation is very rapid (e.g. heart rate > 150), it may be difficult to distinguish from SVT because at a very fast rate it may appear to be a regular rhythm. If at a glance the rhythm appears to be regular, turn the volume up on the cardiac monitor. If the rhythm is irregular, it will become apparent from the sound.

Hallmark of atrial fib.: Irregularly irregular rhythm

Atrial flutter

Example

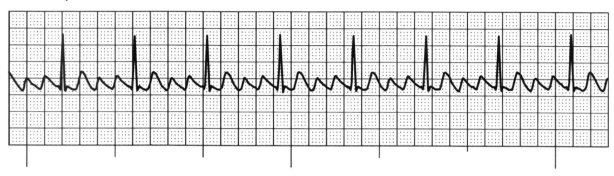

☐	Rate:	The heart rate in atrial flutter is usually fast. It may be normal or slow with drug therapy.
☐	P waves	In atrial flutter the *P waves* have a classical *saw-tooth* appearance. The atria fire at a rate of 200-350/minute.
☐	PR:	N/A
☐	QRS:	Usually narrow.
☐	Ratio	The AV node blocks many of the atrial impulses, thus protecting the ventricles from being overwhelmed. The ratio may be 2:1, 3:1, 4:1, or vary from beat to beat, particularly if the patient is on antiarrhythmics.
☐	Rhythm:	Usually regular.

Describe this rhythm: _____

_____

The saw-tooth results from a rapid firing of ectopic impulses from one of the atria. The AV node serves to protect the ventricles by limiting the number of impulses getting through. It allows every second, third or fourth impulse to conduct to the ventricles resulting in a 2:1, 3:1, or 4:1 conduction).

When every *second* impulse conducts through to the ventricles, the heart rate may be so fast (typically HR 150) that it makes atrial flutter indistinguishable from SVT. Increasing the vagal tone (e.g. valsalva maneuver) may slow conduction through the AV node temporarily and the flutter waves will then appear on the ECG.

Saw-tooth pattern

1st Degree AV Block

Example

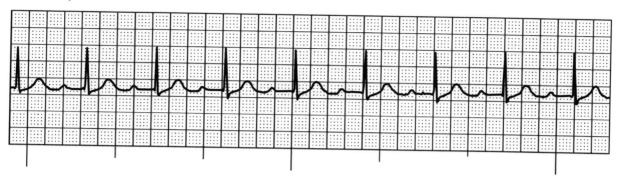

☐	**Rate:**	The heart rate may slow, normal or fast.
☐	**P waves**	Are present and upright in leads I, II and III.
☐	**PR:**	*The P-R interval is greater than 0.20 second.* *The P-R interval is constant.*
☐	**QRS:**	Is usually narrow (< 0.12 second).
☐	**Ratio:**	One P wave per QRS (1:1).
☐	**Rhythm:**	Regular

Describe this rhythm: _____

1st Degree AV block is a benign rhythm distinguished by a prolonged and consistent P-R interval.

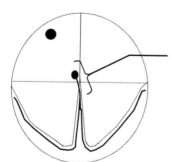

Don't worry. I'll let all of you sinus impulses through, I'm just getting a little older and it takes me a little longer than it use to.

P-R interval greater than 0.20 sec.

2nd Degree AV Block, Type I (Wenkebach)

Example

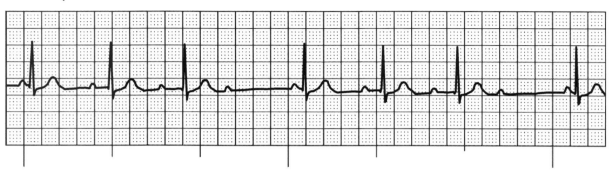

☐ Rate: Generally slow to normal.

☐ P waves Are present and upright in leads I, II, and III.
In Wenkebach you will see dropped beats, or P waves that stand alone.

☐ PR: The P-R interval becomes increasingly prolonged until a beat is dropped. The change in P-R interval may be very subtle. Look at the P-R interval before and after the dropped beat. **The one before will be longer than the one after.**

☐ QRS: Are usually narrow (< 0.12 second).

☐ Ratio 1:1 in the underlying rhythm and 2: 1 where the dropped beat occurs.

☐ Rhythm: Regularly irregular.

Describe this rhythm: _____

In Wenkebach the P-R interval gets progressively longer (refractory period of the AV node gets longer) until a beat is blocked and you see a P wave standing alone. The example above is one in which the cycle of dropped beats occurs frequently. Wenkebach may not always be so obvious; i.e. dropped beats may occur far less often. Therefore, when you see a P wave that stands alone, look at the P-R interval before and after the dropped beat. The P-R interval before the dropped beat will be longer than the P-R interval after the dropped beat. This is Wenckebach signature.

2nd Degree AV block, Type II

Example

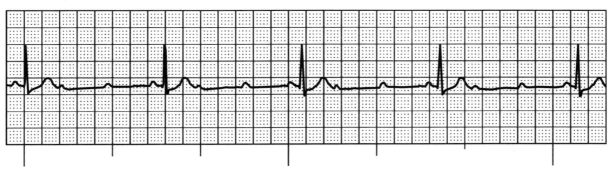

☐	Rate:	*Generally slow.* P waves may fire at a normal rate but only every second or third one is able to conduct through the diseased or ischemic AV node.
☐	P waves	Are present and upright in leads I, II and III.
☐	PR:	Where there are P waves associated with QRS complexes *the P-R interval will be constant.*
☐	QRS:	Are usually narrow (< 0.12 second).
☐	Ratio	*There is usually a fixed ratio of 2:1, 3:1 or rarely 4:1.* Less commonly, patients may have intermittent 2nd Degree AV block Type II with a variable ratio of Ps to QRSs.
☐	Rhythm:	*Usually regular* unless there is intermittent block and/or the ratio varies.

Describe this rhythm: _____

_____

In most cases of 2nd Degree Type II AV block the heart rate is bradycardic and the ratio of P waves to QRS complexes is constant. In all cases the P waves that are associated with QRS complexes will have a consistent P-R interval.

Because the heart rate is generally quite slow with this type of block it **can be** a potentially **life-threatening** rhythm that requires immediate attention.

Slow, regular rhythm with 2 or 3 P waves per QRS (usually)

3rd Degree AV block (complete heart block)

Example

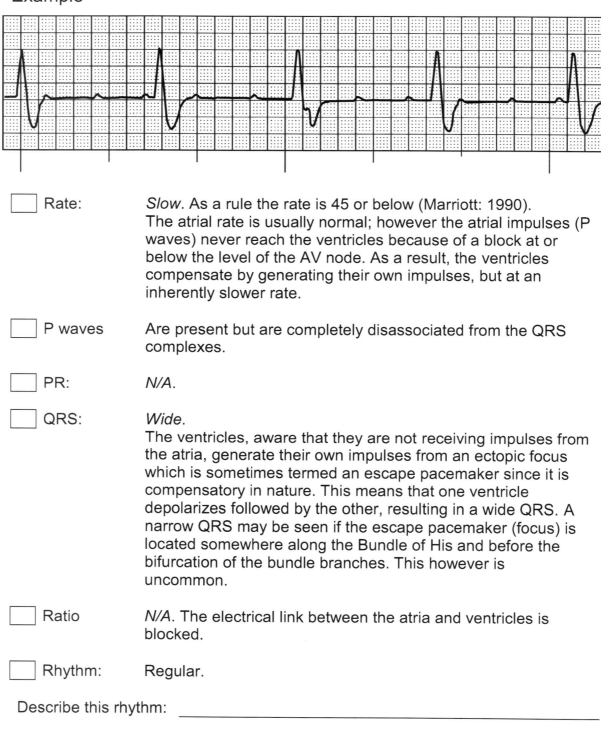

	Rate:	*Slow*. As a rule the rate is 45 or below (Marriott: 1990). The atrial rate is usually normal; however the atrial impulses (P waves) never reach the ventricles because of a block at or below the level of the AV node. As a result, the ventricles compensate by generating their own impulses, but at an inherently slower rate.
	P waves	Are present but are completely disassociated from the QRS complexes.
	PR:	*N/A*.
	QRS:	*Wide*. The ventricles, aware that they are not receiving impulses from the atria, generate their own impulses from an ectopic focus which is sometimes termed an escape pacemaker since it is compensatory in nature. This means that one ventricle depolarizes followed by the other, resulting in a wide QRS. A narrow QRS may be seen if the escape pacemaker (focus) is located somewhere along the Bundle of His and before the bifurcation of the bundle branches. This however is uncommon.
	Ratio	*N/A*. The electrical link between the atria and ventricles is blocked.
	Rhythm:	Regular.

Describe this rhythm: _____

3rd Degree AV block continued...

Whenever you see a slow, wide complex (meaning wide QRS) rhythm in which there are also P waves present, your first assumption should be that it is 3rd Degree AV block. At that point you begin looking for evidence to support or refute that assumption. In 3rd Degree AV block there is AV dissociation. P waves will be equidistant and will "march through" the rhythm. This means that the P waves will march along completely independent of the QRS complexes. Where the P waves are buried in the QRS you will often see an alteration in the QRS morphology indicating that the P wave is buried there.

Look for the following:

| Why is the QRS wide ? |

1. **Slow wide (usually) complex regular rhythm**
2. **P waves "marching through" (AV dissociation)**
3. **Alteration in the QRS morphology where the P is buried in the QRS**

Physical findings:

Look for irregular cannon A waves: Since the atria and ventricles beat independently, at times the atria will | Because the focus is in one of the ventricles ! | contract against closed AV valves. This causes a back-flow of blood into the jugular veins and the so-called "cannon A waves". Look at the jugular veins for occasional expansive pulsation.

Hemodynamics:

How the patient presents hemodynamically with a 3rd Degree AV block depends on a number of factors including:

1. How slow the heart rate is.
2. The patient's age.
3. The condition of the patient's heart.
4. Other stressors or co-existing disease(s).

The patient may be hemodynamically stable, unstable or may be in imminent risk of cardiac arrest. Generally however, this is a low (cardiac) output rhythm that is or has the potential to be life-threatening and dictates immediate attention and constant supervision regardless of the patient's initial clinical presentation.

Idioventricular rhythm

Example

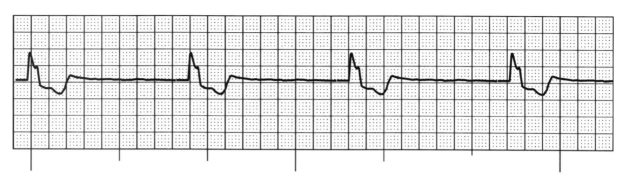

☐ Rate: Slow. Generally 20-40.
             The cells of the ventricles, when put in the position of having to
             generate impulses, do so at an inherently slower pace. Rates
             >40 and <100 are indicative of an accelerated idioventricular
             rhythm or AIVR.

☐ P waves   Absent.

☐ PR: N/A

☐ QRS: Wide. $\geq$ 0.12 second.

☐ Ratio   N/A

☐ Rhythm: Regular.

How to describe this rhythm: _____

An idioventricular rhythm, or ventricular escape rhythm as it is otherwise known, is
a rhythm that originates from an impulse in the ventricles when higher pacemaker
sites have failed.

Hemodynamics:

Like a 3rd Degree AV block, how the patient presents clinically depends on how
slow the heart rate is, the patient's age and the condition of their heart, and the
presence of other stresses or co-existing conditions. This is an inherently unstable
rhythm and may require immediate attention.

Slow, regular, wide complex rhythm - No P waves

Premature ventricular complex (PVC)

Example

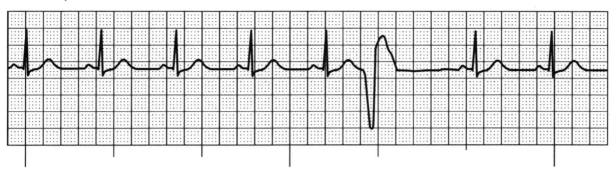

☐	Rate:	The underlying rhythm may be slow, normal or fast.
☐	P waves:	*No P wave preceding the PVC.* PVCs are sometimes conducted into the atria, producing a retrograde P wave.
☐	PR:	N/A.
☐	QRS:	Wide & bizarre. The QRS of a PVC will be at least 0.12 second and is usually 0.14 second or greater. The PVC may also be opposite in deflection from the QRSs in the underlying rhythm.
☐	Ratio:	N/A where the PVC occurs.
☐	Rhythm:	The underlying rhythm may be regular except where disrupted by the PVC (s), or the underlying rhythm may be irregular if it is atrial fib. or some other irregular rhythm.

How to describe this rhythm: _____

_____

Your first task is to identify the underlying rhythm using a step by step approach. Then look at the FLBs (funny looking beats) and identify them using the following criteria.

1. Do they occur early, or before the next expected beat?
2. Are they wide (≥ 0.12 sec.) and bizarre in shape compared to the other QRSs?
3. If the wide and bizarre QRS is opposite in deflection from the QRSs in the underlying rhythm (example above), this confirms that it is indeed a PVC.

A PVC results when an impulse is generated from an ectopic focus somewhere in one of the ventricles. It occurs prematurely, or before the next expected beat, and is often, but not always, followed by a **compensatory pause.** This means that the distance between the preceding beat and the beat following the PVC is equal to two cardiac cycles.

The reason a PVC is wide and bizarre is because the impulse is generated in one of the ventricles. Therefore, instead of the impulse descending the Bundle of His and both bundle branches simultaneously as it does in normally conducted beats, the wave of depolarization begins in one ventricle then spreads to the other.

PVCs arise from parts of the ventricle (s) that are scarred from previous infarctions, ischemic regions, or from irritation caused by caffeine, nicotine, lack of sleep, anxiety, etc.

SOME EXAMPLES OF PATTERNS SEEN WITH PVCs

Multiform PVCs: Originating from more than one focus or from the same focus but where the direction of the initial wave of depolarization differs with each impulse. The term **polymorphic PVCs** is also used to describe this.

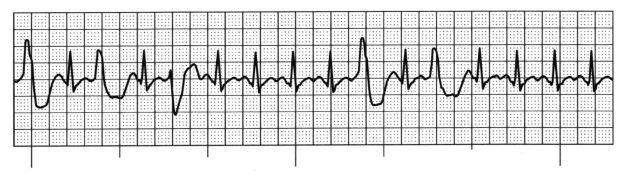

Bigeminy: A PVC every second beat.

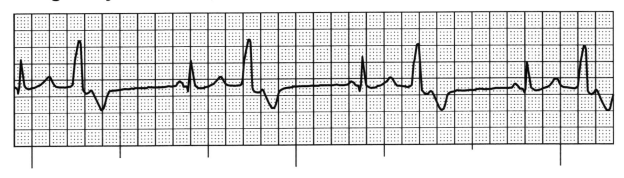

Trigeminy: A PVC every third beat.

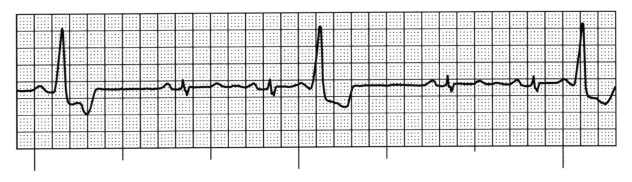

Quadrigeminy: A PVC every fourth beat.

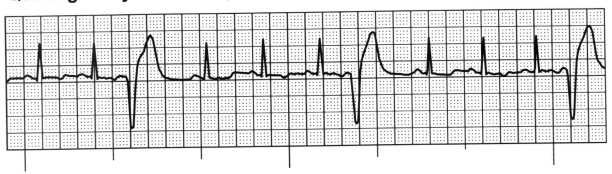

Couplet: Two ventricular ectopic beats that are side by side.

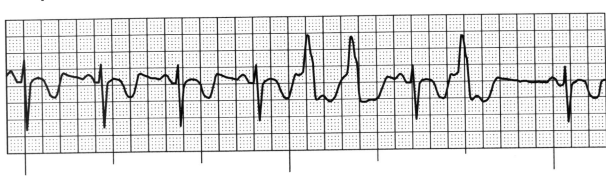

Ventricular tachycardia (V. tach. or V.T.)

Example

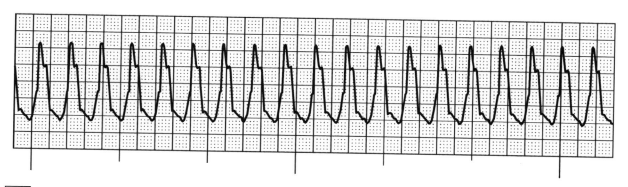

	Rate:	Usually between 120 - 250. Rates greater than 250/ minute are considered ventricular flutter.
	P waves	AV dissociation is present in approximately 50 % of all V.T.s and when present, is diagnostic - Ps march independent of QRSs. A discernible P wave preceding each QRS is suggestive of a supraventricular tachycardia that is aberrantly conducted.
	PR:	N/A
	QRS:	Always wide. i.e. $\geq$ 0.12 second. Usually $\geq$ 0.14 second
	Ratio	N/A. Look for AV dissociation.
	Rhythm:	Usually regular unless it's a multiform (polymorphic) V.T.

Describe this rhythm: _____

If you're confronted with a wide complex tachycardia of uncertain origin, it's likely V. Tach. it should be treated as such. If the patient is stable, then a 12 lead ECG can be obtained to help confirm the type of tachycardia.

* SVT with aberrant conduction is one rhythm that will sometimes mimic V.T.

Ventricular tachycardia is defined as three or more ventricular ectopic beats in a row (at a rate $\geq$ 120/min.). VT may occur in short runs or it may be sustained.

Fast, regular (usually), wide complex rhythm

ABERRANT CONDUCTION
another cause for a wide QRS

Aberrancy means to stray from the normal path or to wander. In electrocardiographic terms it means that the impulse(s) generated from above the ventricles descends through the AV node and bundle of His and is then blocked in one of the bundle branches or the smaller branches coming off of the left bundle branch. By definition the term applies only to transient conduction defects. However, it is used liberally by many, though perhaps not correctly, to describe all supraventricular beats or rhythms in which the QRS is 0.12 second or greater.

Example

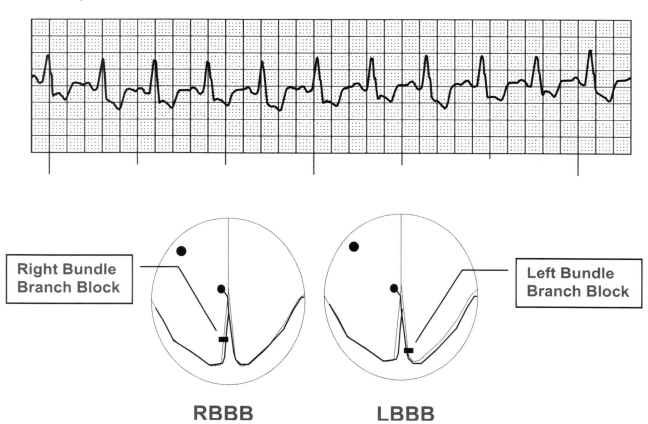

RBBB   **LBBB**

A presence of a bundle branch block is the most common cause of a wide QRS in a supraventricular rhythm.

There are also a number of other causes of supraventricular rhythms with a wide QRS. These include fascicular blocks, drug effect, electrolyte imbalance, etc

Ventricular fibrillation (V. fib. or V.F.)

Example

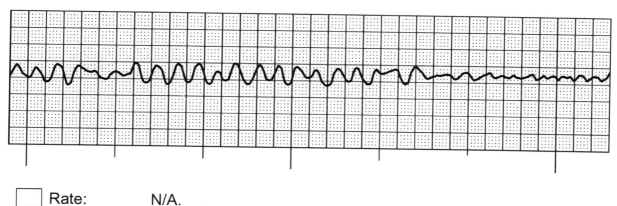

☐ Rate: N/A.

☐ P waves N/A.

☐ PR: N/A.

☐ QRS: N/A.

☐ Ratio N/A.

☐ Rhythm: N/A.

Describe this rhythm: _____

The patient in V.F. is clinically dead or vital signs absent.

The ECG pattern in V.F. is a reflection of electrical chaos within the ventricles. Multiple competing sites (foci) within the ventricles generate impulses. Hundreds of aimless waves of depolarization collide with one another canceling each other out. From a *mechanical* perspective the result is a quivering mass of ventricular myocardium.

SHOCK ME !

Asystole

Example

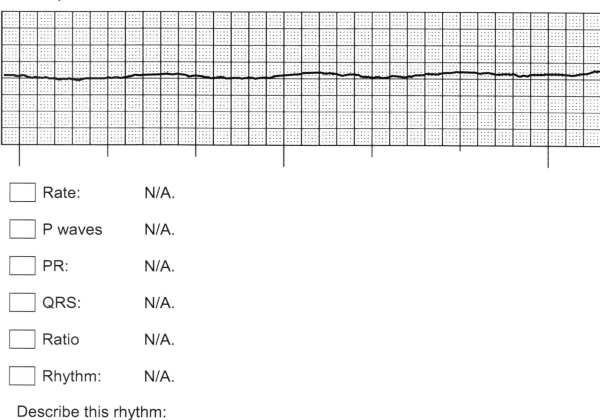

	Rate:	N/A.
☐	P waves	N/A.
☐	PR:	N/A.
☐	QRS:	N/A.
☐	Ratio	N/A.
☐	Rhythm:	N/A.

Describe this rhythm: _____

The patient in asystole is clinically dead or vital signs absent.

Asystole appears on the monitor as a *virtually* flat line. There is a complete absence of electrical and mechanical activity.

Asystole may also be the sequelae of a bradycardia that deteriorates, or the result of excessive vagal stimulation. I like to refer to Asystole as *the mother of all bradycardias.*

V.F. will also eventually deteriorate into asystole over time if it is not defibrillated.

One should always confirm asystole by checking for a pulse, ensure all the leads are properly connected, check the rhythm in two leads, and turn up the ECG size on the monitor to verify that it's not fine V.F. masquerading as asystole. Note: a *perfectly* flat line is more likely caused by a lead disconnection.

Flat-line on the ECG

Pulseless electrical activity (P.E.A.)
Formally called: Electromechanical activity (EMD)

Example

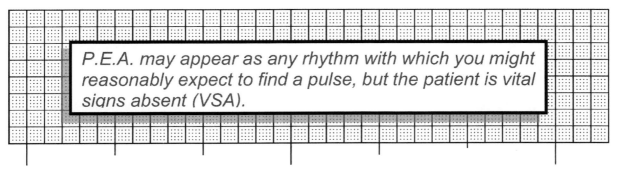

P.E.A. may appear as any rhythm with which you might reasonably expect to find a pulse, but the patient is vital signs absent (VSA).

The patient with P.E.A. is clinically dead or vital signs absent.

P.E.A. describes the presence of some form of cardiac rhythm in a patient who is apneic and pulseless (a non-perfusing rhythm).

The rhythm on the monitor may be anything from a sinus tachycardia to an idioventricular rhythm. This is why it is that you assess and treat the patient and not focus on the cardiac monitor. Part of the patient assessment and treatment for P.E.A. entails commencing CPR immediately and beginning the search for the underlying cause.

The following are some of the causes of P.E.A.:

5 Hs:
Hypovolemia,
Hypoxia,
Hydrogen Ion (acidosis),
Hyper/hypokalemia,
Hypothermia

5 Ts:
Tablets (drug overdose),
Tamponade,
Tension pneumothorax,
Thrombosis (coronary – i.e. massive MI),
Thrombosis (pulmonary embolism or PE).

Organized ECG rhythm – but patient is unresponsive, apneic & pulseless

ARTIFACT
EXAMPLES

Somatic tremor

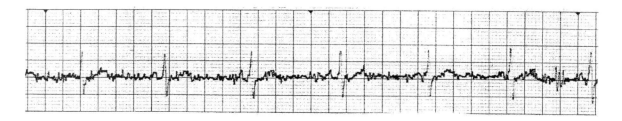

Description

In addition to sensing the heart's electrical activity, cardiac monitors will also sense skeletal muscle activity when a patient is moving or is tense. The signal from skeletal muscle is not as strong as that of cardiac muscle so it does not usually obscure QRS complexes. It may however completely disrupt the base line of the ECG tracing, making P waves indiscernible.

Causes

Patient movement - nervousness, fear, apprehension - shivering - Parkinson's disease - etc.

To correct

Explain the procedure and reassure the patient that it is painless - keep the patient warm - if the patient suffers from tremors from Parkinson's disease, have the patient place their hands under their buttocks and support their head and legs with pillows - check for broken or frayed cables.

Alternating current (60 cycle) interference

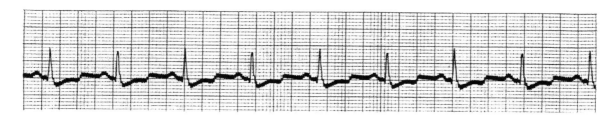

Description

60 cycle interference is caused by a leakage in electrical power. It is easily identified by its uniform fine sawtooth appearance along the baseline.

Causes

Nearby electrical appliances; e.g.. mechanical ventilator, suction unit, electrical bed, etc - improper grounding; e.g.. third prong on the monitor plug missing or broken, ground electrode not connected to the patient - concealed wiring - patient touching electrode or metal parts of the bed while the ECG recording is taking place.

To correct

If possible, disconnect nearby appliance (s). - Make sure the monitor is grounded with a three prong plug. - Make sure the ground plug is attached to the patient. - Make sure the patient is not touching metal parts of the bed.

Points to remember⋎⎯⎮⎯⋏⎯⎮⎯⋏⎯⎮⎯⋏⎯⎮⎯⋏⎯

- Use a *Step by Step* approach.

- Calculate heart rate first and always include the heart rate in your description of the rhythm.

- Look for P waves. Is there a P wave associated with each QRS ? If so, this tells you that there is AV synchrony, or that the electrical link between the atria and the ventricles is intact.

- The morphology (shape) of the QRS and T waves is not important where *rhythm* interpretation is concerned; so don't be overly worried if they are deflected negatively instead of positively. What is important is the QRS duration. **Normal QRS duration is < 0.12 second**. A QRS of ≥ 0.12 second is considered wide.

- In the normal rhythm, the ratio of P waves to QRSs is 1:1. A greater ratio than 1:1 indicates that not all impulses generated in the atria are able to conduct through to the ventricles. In 2nd degree AV block types I and II for example, the AV node and/or perinodal tissue has a longer than normal refractory period. On the other hand, in atrial flutter the AV node may be healthy, however impulses are generated too quickly for the AV node to accommodate them all. Therefore, some reach the AV node while it's still in its normal refractory period and get blocked.

- **Normal P-R interval is 0.12 - 0.20 second**.

Remember: Use the *Step by Step* approach.

Analyze each ECG carefully. It's fine to start with a hunch, but then follow it up with a step by step approach to gather the necessary evidence that will lead you to the correct conclusion. If you start out certain that you *know* what the rhythm is, chances are you'll look only for evidence to support what you *think* is the correct interpretation and you'll miss other important clues.

So keep an open mind and remember that there are pearls and pitfalls along the journey to ECG interpretation.

Warning: After you've had some experience interpreting ECGs it's easy to become complacent and fall into the habit of interpreting ECGs based on "pattern recognition"; i.e.. having seen dozens of similar ECG patterns in the past, "this EGG must be..." This approach often results in embarrassing and potentially serious mistakes.

Note: The answers for the following ECG strips can be found in Appendix A at the end of the book.

STRIP # 1

RATE: _____

P WAVES: _____

P-R: _____

QRS: _____ RATIO (# of P to QRS): _____

RHYTHM: _____

Your interpretation: _____

_____

STRIP # 2

RATE: _____

P WAVES: _____

P-R: _____

QRS: _____ RATIO (# of P to QRS): _____

RHYTHM: _____

Your interpretation: _____

_____

STRIP # 3

RATE: _____

P WAVES: _____

P-R: _____

QRS: _____ RATIO (# of P to QRS): _____

RHYTHM: _____

Your interpretation: _____

STRIP # 4

RATE: _____

P WAVES: _____

P-R: _____

QRS: _____ RATIO (# of P to QRS): _____

RHYTHM: _____

Your interpretation: _____

STRIP # 5

RATE: _____

P WAVES: _____

P-R: _____

QRS: _____   RATIO (# of P to QRS): _____

RHYTHM: _____

Your interpretation: _____

_____

STRIP # 6

RATE: _____

P WAVES: _____

P-R: _____

QRS: _____   RATIO (# of P to QRS): _____

RHYTHM: _____

Your interpretation: _____

_____

STRIP # 7

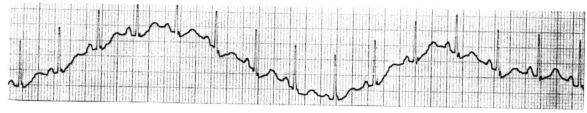

RATE: _____

P WAVES: _____

P-R: _____

QRS: _____   RATIO (# of P to QRS): _____

RHYTHM: _____

Your interpretation: _____

STRIP # 8

RATE: _____

P WAVES: _____

P-R: _____

QRS: _____   RATIO (# of P to QRS): _____

RHYTHM: _____

Your interpretation: _____

STRIP # 9

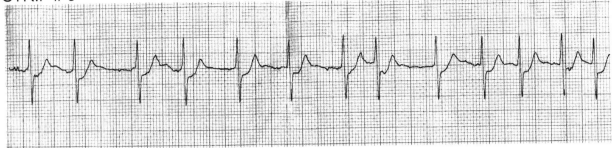

RATE: _____

P WAVES: _____

P-R: _____

QRS: _____ RATIO (# of P to QRS): _____

RHYTHM: _____

Your interpretation: _____

STRIP # 10

RHYTHM STRIP: II
25 mm/sec; 1 cm/mV

RATE: _____

P WAVES: _____

P-R: _____

QRS: _____ RATIO (# of P to QRS): _____

RHYTHM: _____

Your interpretation: _____

STRIP # 11

RATE: _____

P WAVES: _____

P-R: _____

QRS: _____ RATIO (# of P to QRS): _____

RHYTHM: _____

Your interpretation: _____

STRIP # 12

RATE: _____

P WAVES: _____

P-R: _____

QRS: _____ RATIO (# of P to QRS): _____

RHYTHM: _____

Your interpretation: _____

STRIP # 13

RATE: _____

P WAVES: _____

P-R: _____

QRS: _____   RATIO (# of P to QRS): _____

RHYTHM: _____

Your interpretation: _____

STRIP # 14

RATE: _____

P WAVES: _____

P-R: _____

QRS: _____   RATIO (# of P to QRS): _____

RHYTHM: _____

Your interpretation: _____

STRIP # 15

RATE: _____

P WAVES: _____

P-R: _____

QRS: _____   RATIO (# of P to QRS): _____

RHYTHM: _____

Your interpretation: _____

STRIP # 16

RATE: _____

P WAVES: _____

P-R: _____

QRS: _____   RATIO (# of P to QRS): _____

RHYTHM: _____

Your interpretation: _____

STRIP # 17

RATE: _____

P WAVES: _____

P-R: _____

QRS: _____ RATIO (# of P to QRS): _____

RHYTHM: _____

Your interpretation: _____

STRIP # 18

RATE: _____

P WAVES: _____

P-R: _____

QRS: _____ RATIO (# of P to QRS): _____

RHYTHM: _____

Your interpretation: _____

STRIP # 19

RATE: _____

P WAVES: _____

P-R: _____

QRS: _____   RATIO (# of P to QRS): _____

RHYTHM: _____

Your interpretation: _____

STRIP # 20

RATE: _____

P WAVES: _____

P-R: _____

QRS: _____   RATIO (# of P to QRS): _____

RHYTHM: _____

Your interpretation: _____

STRIP # 21

RATE: _____

P WAVES: _____

P-R: _____

QRS: _____   RATIO (# of P to QRS): _____

RHYTHM: _____

Your interpretation: _____

STRIP # 22

RATE: _____

P WAVES: _____

P-R: _____

QRS: _____   RATIO (# of P to QRS): _____

RHYTHM: _____

Your interpretation: _____

STRIP # 23

RATE: _____

P WAVES: _____

P-R: _____

QRS: _____ RATIO (# of P to QRS): _____

RHYTHM: _____

Your interpretation: _____

STRIP # 24

RATE: _____

P WAVES: _____

P-R: _____

QRS: _____ RATIO (# of P to QRS): _____

RHYTHM: _____

Your interpretation: _____

STRIP # 25

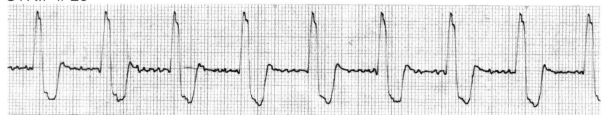

RATE: _____

P WAVES: _____

P-R: _____

QRS: _____ RATIO (# of P to QRS): _____

RHYTHM: _____

Your interpretation: _____

STRIP # 26

RATE: _____

P WAVES: _____

P-R: _____

QRS: _____ RATIO (# of P to QRS): _____

RHYTHM: _____

Your interpretation: _____

STRIP # 27

RHYTHM STRIP:]]
25 mm/sec; 1 cm/mV

RATE: _____

P WAVES: _____

P-R: _____

QRS: _____   RATIO (# of P to QRS): _____

RHYTHM: _____

Your interpretation: _____

_____

STRIP # 28

RATE: _____

P WAVES: _____

P-R: _____

QRS: _____   RATIO (# of P to QRS): _____

RHYTHM: _____

Your interpretation: _____

STRIP # 29

RATE: _____

P WAVES: _____

P-R: _____

QRS: _____ RATIO (# of P to QRS): _____

RHYTHM: _____

Your interpretation: _____

STRIP # 30

RATE: _____

P WAVES: _____

P-R: _____

QRS: _____ RATIO (# of P to QRS): _____

RHYTHM: _____

Your interpretation: _____

STRIP # 31

RATE: _____

P WAVES: _____

P-R: _____

QRS: _____   RATIO (# of P to QRS): _____

RHYTHM: _____

Your interpretation: _____

STRIP # 32

RATE: _____

P WAVES: _____

P-R: _____

QRS: _____   RATIO (# of P to QRS): _____

RHYTHM: _____

Your interpretation: _____

STRIP # 33

PHYSIO-CONTROL®   P/N 804700

RATE: _____

P WAVES: _____

P-R: _____

QRS: _____   RATIO (# of P to QRS): _____

RHYTHM: _____

Your interpretation: _____

_____

STRIP # 34

NO PHY 09-10419

RATE: _____

P WAVES: _____

P-R: _____

QRS: _____   RATIO (# of P to QRS): _____

RHYTHM: _____

Your interpretation: _____

_____

STRIP # 35

RATE: _____

P WAVES: _____

P-R: _____

QRS: _____   RATIO (# of P to QRS): _____

RHYTHM: _____

Your interpretation: _____

STRIP # 36

RATE: _____

P WAVES: _____

P-R: _____

QRS: _____   RATIO (# of P to QRS): _____

RHYTHM: _____

Your interpretation: _____

STRIP # 37

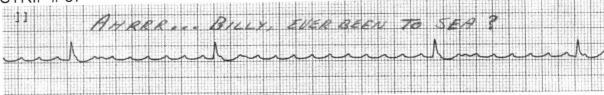

AHRRR... BILLY, EVER BEEN TO SEA ?

RATE: _____

P WAVES: _____

P-R: _____

QRS: _____   RATIO (# of P to QRS): _____

RHYTHM: _____

Your interpretation: _____

_____

STRIP # 38

RATE: _____

P WAVES: _____

P-R: _____

QRS: _____   RATIO (# of P to QRS): _____

RHYTHM: _____

Your interpretation: _____

_____

STRIP # 39 (2 y/o who collapsed after inhaling chlorine gas)

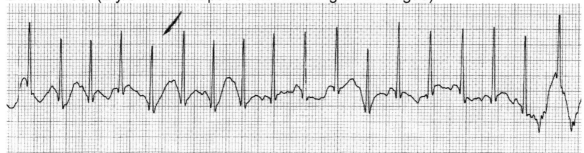

RATE: _____

P WAVES: _____

P-R: _____

QRS: _____ RATIO (# of P to QRS): _____

RHYTHM: _____

Your interpretation: _____

STRIP # 40

RATE: _____

P WAVES: _____

P-R: _____

QRS: _____ RATIO (# of P to QRS): _____

RHYTHM: _____

Your interpretation: _____

REFERENCES

1. Tintinalli, J.E., et al: **Emergency Medicine: A Comprehensive Study Guide.** Sixth Edition. New York: McGraw Hill, 2004.

BIBLIOGRAPHY

Boudreau Conover, M.: **Understanding Electrocardiography. Eighth Edition**. St. Louis: Mosby, 2003.

Dubin, D.: **Rapid Interpretation of E.K.G.s, Sixth Edition**. Tampa: Cover Publishing Company, 2000.

Marriott, H.J.L.: **Pearls & Pitfalls in Electrocardiography. Second Edition**. Malvern: Lea & Febiger, 1998.

Tintinalli, J.E., et al: **Emergency Medicine: A Comprehensive Study Guide**. Sixth Edition. New York: McGraw Hill, 2004.

Walraven, G.: **Basic Arrhythmias**. Fifth Edition *Revised*. New Jersey: Prentice Hall Inc., 2005.

Wellens, J.J.H., and Conover, M.B.: **The ECG in Emergency Decision Making. Second Edition**. Philadelphia: W.B. Saunders, 2005.

Appendix A
ECG Answers (for further discussion, you can contact me at: rob.t@sympatico.ca)

Strip #1 (p. 85) Rate: ~80 / 180-200 P waves: present initially P-R: ~0.16 Ratio: 1:1 initially QRS: narrow Rhythm: regular Interpretation: normal sinus rhythm with a bout of PSVT with a heart rate of ~ 180-200	**Strip #2 (p. 85)** Rate: 100-120 (there is no right or wrong answer, just a range P waves: not discernable P-R: N/A Ratio: N/A QRS: narrow Rhythm: irregularly irregular Interpretation: Atrial fibrillation with a ventricular response between 100 and 120
Strip #3 (p. 86) Rate: ~30 P waves: present and upright P-R: 0.16 second Ratio: 1:1 QRS: 0.10 second - narrow Rhythm: regular Interpretation: sinus bradycardia with a heart rate of ~30/min.	**Strip #4 (p.86)** Rate: ~40 P waves: inverted P-R: 0.04 - 0.06 short Ratio: 1:1 QRS: 0.08 second - narrow Rhythm: regular Interpretation: junctional rhythm with a heart rate of ~40/min.
Strip #5 (p.87) Rate: ~72 P waves: present - one has a different shape P-R: 0.14 second / normal Ratio: 1:1 QRS: 0.08 second / narrow Rhythm: mostly regular Interpretation: normal sinus rhythm with a heart rate of ~ 70/min with one PAC	**Strip #6 (p.87)** Rate: ~80-85 P waves: flutter waves (at 250-300/min - not important to document) P-R: N/A Ratio: variable ratio QRS: narrow Rhythm: regular Interpretation: Atrial flutter with a heart rate of ~120 and a variable conduction ratio
Strip #7 (p.88) Rate: ~130 P waves: Present & upright P-R: 0.16 second Ratio: 1:1 QRS: narrow Rhythm: regular Interpretation: sinus tachycardia with a heart rate of 130 bpm	**Strip #8 (p.88)** Rate: ~42 P waves: present P-R: 0.24 second Ratio: 1:1 QRS: narrow Rhythm: irregular Interpretation: sinus bradycardia with a sinus arrest (sinus pause) that lasts ~ 3 seconds (there is also a 1° AV block)
Strip #9 (p.89) Rate: ~80-100 P waves: not discernable P-R: N/A Ratio: N/A QRS: narrow Rhythm: irregularly irregular Interpretation: atrial fibrillation with a ventricular response of 80-100	**Strip #10 (p.89)** Rate: ~85 P waves: present and upright P-R: 0.18 second - normal Ratio: 1:1 QRS: probably narrow (ST elevation present) Rhythm: regular Interpretation: normal sinus rhythm with a heart rate of 85 (note: because there is marked ST elevation, a 12 Lead ECG should be done)
Strip #11 (p.90) Rate: ~30 P waves: present and upright P-R: 0.14-0.16 second Ratio: 1:1 QRS: narrow Rhythm: regular Interpretation: sinus bradycardia with a heart rate of 30 and a single PVC	**Strip #12 (p.90)** Rate: ~210 P waves: not discernable P-R: N/A Ratio: N/A QRS: narrow Rhythm: regular Interpretation: SVT with a heart rate of 210

Strip #13 (p.91)	Strip #14 (p.91)
Rate: ~48 P waves: absent P-R: N/A Ratio: N/A QRS: narrow Rhythm: regular Interpretation: junctional rhythm with a heart rate of ~48 /min.	Rate: ~70 P waves: present & upright P-R: normal (where there are P waves associated with the QRSs) Ratio: 1:1 QRS: narrow Rhythm: irregular Interpretation: NSR with 4 PJCs
Strip #15 (p.92)	**Strip #16 (p.92)**
Rate: ~33 P waves: present & upright P-R: ~ 0.28 second - prolonged Ratio: 2:1 QRS: wide Rhythm: regular Interpretation: 2° AV block type II with a heart rate of 33 and a 2:1 conduction ratio	Rate: ~120 P waves: present & upright P-R: 0.16 second Ratio: 1:1 QRS: narrow Rhythm: irregular Interpretation: sinus tachycardia with frequent multiform PVCs
Strip #17 (p.93)	**Strip #18 (p.93)**
Rate: ~58 P waves: present & upright P-R: 0.22 second - prolonged Ratio: 1:1 QRS: wide Rhythm: regular Interpretation: sinus bradycardia with a heart rate of ~58 and aberrant conduction	Rate: ~35 P waves: absent P-R: N/A Ratio: N/A QRS: wide Rhythm: regular Interpretation: idioventricular rhythm with a heart rate of ~35/min.
Strip #19 (p.94)	**Strip #20 (p.94)**
Rate: ~40 P waves: present P-R: normal Ratio: N/A – P waves not related to QRSs QRS: narrow Rhythm: regular Interpretation: 3rd Degree AV block with a heart rate of 40	Rate: ~60-100 P waves: flutter waves P-R: N/A Ratio: varies QRS: narrow Rhythm: irregular Interpretation: atrial flutter with a heart rate of ~ 60-100 with a variable conduction ratio
Strip #21 (p.95)	**Strip #22 (p.95)**
Rate: ~25 P waves: present P-R: not associated with the QRSs Ratio: N/A QRS: wide Rhythm: regular Interpretation: 3rd Degree AV block with a heart rate of ~ 25	Rate: ~130 P waves: present in the underlying rhythm - none associated with the FLBs P-R: normal Ratio: 1:1 QRS: narrow - wide in the FLBs Rhythm: irregular Interpretation: sinus tachycardia with a heart rate of 130, with a couplet and a short run of V. Tach.
Strip #23 (p.96)	**Strip #24 (p.96)**
Rate: ~85 P waves: present P-R: 0.16 second Ratio: 1:1 QRS: wide Rhythm: regular Interpretation: sinus rhythm with a heart rate of 85 with aberrant conduction	Rate: ~210 initially P waves: absent P-R: N/A Ratio: N/A QRS: wide Rhythm: regular - chaos Interpretation: V. Tach. that deteriorates into V.F.

Strip #25 (p.97)	Strip #26 (p.97)
Rate: ~75 P waves: not discernable P-R: N/A Ratio: N/A QRS: wide Rhythm: regular Interpretation: accelerated idioventricular rhythm with a heart rate of ~75/min. Note: this cannot be atrial fibrillation because it is regular	Rate: ~72 P waves: present P-R: increasing in length Ratio: varies from 1:1 to 2:1 QRS: narrow Rhythm: irregular Interpretation: 2° AV block type I with a heart rate of ~72
Strip #27 (p.98)	**Strip #28 (p.98)**
Rate: ~130 P waves: present P-R: 0.16 second Ratio: 1:1 QRS: wide & bizarre Rhythm: regular Interpretation: sinus tachycardia with a heart rate of ~130	Rate: ~34 P waves: present P-R: consistent with each P wave that's followed by a QRS Ratio: 3:1 QRS: narrow Rhythm: regular Interpretation: 2° AV block type II with a heart rate of ~34
Strip #29 (p.99)	**Strip #30 (p.99)**
Rate: ~210 P waves: absent P-R: N/A Ratio: N/A QRS: narrow in the underlying rhythm Rhythm: irregular Interpretation: SVT with a heart rate of 210 with frequent (5) uniform PVCs	Rate: ~100-150 P waves: not discernable P-R: N/A Ratio: N/A QRS: narrow Rhythm: irregularly irregular Interpretation: atrial fibrillation with a ventricular response of ~120-1
`Strip #31 (p.100)	Strip #32 (p.100)
Interpretation: 3° AV block with a heart rate of ~ 20/min.	Interpretation: ventricular standstill or asystole - this is what can happen when you administer an antiarrhythmic to someone with a 3° AV block; you knock out the focus that keeps the patient alive.....this looks bad on your resume! This would be treated like asystole, except that it has a better prognosis than asystole because it suggest a fresh cardiac arrest.
Strip #33 (p.101)	Strip #34 (p.101)
Interpretation: agonal rhythm...AKA "dying heart"	Interpretation: torsade de Pointes
Strip #35 (p.102)	Strip #36 (p.102)
Interpretation: dual chamber paced rhythm with a heart rate of 75 (note pacemaker - pacer spikes preceding each P wave and each QRS)	Interpretation: Paced rhythm with frequent loss of capture (or intermittent capture failure) heart rate is ~ 40 Note: some beats are paced while other pacer spikes are not followed by a QRS.
Strip #37 (p.103)	Strip #38 (p.103)
Interpretation: atrial flutter with a heart rate less ~ 20 and a variable conduction ratio (this was a case of Digoxin toxicity)	Interpretation: sinus bradycardia with a heart rate of ~40
Strip #39 (p.104)	Strip #40 (p.104)
Interpretation: sinus tachycardia with a heart rate of 150	Interpretation: sinus bradycardia with a heart rate of 58

Printed in Great Britain
by Amazon